International Political Economy Series

General Editor: **Timothy M. Shaw**, Professor of Commonwealth Governance and Development, and Director of the Institute of Commonwealth Studies, School of Advanced Study, University of London

Titles include:

Glenn Adler and Jonny Steinberg (*editors*)
FROM COMRADES TO CITIZENS
The South African Civics Movement and the Transition to Democracy

Glenn Adler and Eddie Webster (*editors*)
TRADE UNIONS AND DEMOCRATIZATION IN SOUTH AFRICA, 1985–1997

Einar Braathen, Morten Bøås and Gutermund Sæther (*editors*)
ETHNICITY KILLS?
The Politics of War, Peace and Ethnicity in Sub-Saharan Africa

Deborah Bräutigam
CHINESE AID AND AFRICAN DEVELOPMENT
Exporting Green Revolution

Gavin Cawthra
SECURING SOUTH AFRICA'S DEMOCRACY
Defence, Development and Security in Transition

Jennifer Clapp
ADJUSTMENT AND AGRICULTURE IN AFRICA
Farmers, the State and the World Bank in Guinea

Neta C. Crawford and Audie Klotz (*editors*)
HOW SANCTIONS WORK
Lessons from South Africa

Staffan Darnolf and Liisa Laakso (*editors*)
TWENTY YEARS OF INDEPENDENCE IN ZIMBABWE
From Liberation to Authoritarianism

Susan Dicklitch
THE ELUSIVE PROMISE OF NGOs IN AFRICA
Lessons from Uganda

Kevin C. Dunn and Timothy M. Shaw (*editors*)
AFRICA'S CHALLENGE TO INTERNATIONAL RELATIONS THEORY

Kenneth Good
THE LIBERAL MODEL AND AFRICA
Elites Against Democracy

Kees Kingma
DEMOBILIZATION IN SUBSAHARAN AFRICA
The Development and Security Impacts

Vijay S. Makhan
ECONOMIC RECOVERY IN AFRICA
The Paradox of Financial Flows

Clever Mumbengegwi (*editor*)
MACROECONOMIC AND STRUCTURAL ADJUSTMENT POLICIES IN
ZIMBABWE

Colleen O'Manique
NEOLIBERALISM AND AIDS CRISIS IN SUB-SAHARAN AFRICA
Globalization's Pandemic

Nana Poku
REGIONALIZATION AND SECURITY IN SOUTHERN AFRICA

Howard Stein, Olu Ajakaiye and Peter Lewis (*editors*)
DEREGULATION AND THE BANKING CRISIS IN NIGERIA
A Comparative Study

Peter Vale, Larry A. Swatuk and Bertil Oden (*editors*)
THEORY, CHANGE AND SOUTHERN AFRICA'S FUTURE

International Political Economy Series
Series Standing Order ISBN 978-0-333-71708-0 hardcover
Series Standing Order ISBN 978-0-333-71110-1 paperback
(*outside North America only*)

You can receive future titles in this series as they are published by placing a
standing order. Please contact your bookseller or, in case of difficulty, write to
us at the address below with your name and address, the title of the series and
one of the ISBNs quoted above.

Customer Services Department, Macmillan Distribution Ltd, Houndmills,
Basingstoke, Hampshire RG21 6XS, England

Neoliberalism and AIDS Crisis in Sub-Saharan Africa

Globalization's Pandemic

Colleen O'Manique
Trent University
Canada

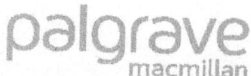

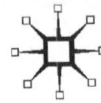
First published 2004 by
PALGRAVE MACMILLAN
Houndmills, Basingstoke, Hampshire RG21 6XS and
175 Fifth Avenue, New York, N.Y. 10010
Companies and representatives throughout the world

PALGRAVE MACMILLAN is the global academic imprint of the Palgrave Macmillan division of St. Martin's Press, LLC and of Palgrave Macmillan Ltd. Macmillan® is a registered trademark in the United States, United Kingdom and other countries. Palgrave is a registered trademark in the European Union and other countries.

ISBN 978-1-4039-2089-8

This book is printed on paper suitable for recycling and made from fully managed and sustained forest sources.

A catalogue record for this book is available from the British Library.

Library of Congress Cataloging-in-Publication Data
O'Manique, Colleen, 1962–.
    Neoliberalism and AIDS crisis in Sub-Saharan Africa : globalization's pandemic / Colleen O'Manique.
        p.   cm. — (International political economy series)
    Includes bibliographical references and index.
    ISBN 978-1-4039-2089-8 (cloth)
    1. AIDS (Disease)—Africa, Sub-Saharan.   2. AIDS (Disease)—Uganda.   3. Africa, Sub-Saharan—Economic policy—Health aspects.   4. Globalization—Health aspects.   I. Title.   II. International political economy series (Palgrave Macmillan (Firm))

RA643.86.A357O46 2004
362.196'9792'00967—dc22
                                                                        2003067400

10   9   8   7   6   5   4   3   2   1
13   12   11   10   09   08   07   06   05   04

Contents

Acknowledgements

The research for this book dates back almost a decade, and the people who assisted me at the beginning of the project are many – thanks to Patricia Stamp, Robert Albritton, Michael Stevenson, Judith Hellman, Kenna Owoh, Jonathan Barker, Richard Stren, and Nakanyike Musisi. In Uganda, Tom Barton, Mary Ssengo, Arnest Wabwire, Narithius Asinguirre, Abbey Nalwanga-Sebina, Harriet Birungi, and Bonnie Keller offered advice and research support, while Agnes Namusisi-Nabakka, and Annette, Nabuwanuka took great care of my daughter. The Makerere Institute of Social Research gave me institutional support, and the International Development Research Centre (Canada) provided me with funding. Juliet O'Manique's support at the beginning of my research was invaluable. Various parts of the book were generously reviewed by Teresa Healy, Katherine Scott, Margaret Barker, Christopher Gombay, John O'Manique, and Erin O'Manique.

Small parts of this book appear in an earlier paper, 'Global Neoliberalism and AIDS Policy: Institutional Responses to Africa's Pandemic', published in *Studies in Political Economy*, May 2004.

At Trent University thanks go to my new colleagues, among them Charmaine Eddy, Judy Pinto, and Erica No1.

The greatest debt is to my mother Patricia O'Manique, my father John O'Manique, to my sisters, and to my daughters Sophie and Claire and my husband Christie, for their constant support along the way.

List of Abbreviations

ACP	AIDS Control Programme
AIDS	Acquired Immune Deficiency Syndrome
AMREF	African Medical and Research Foundation
ARV	Antiretroviral
CHIPS	Community Health Intervention Project against STDs
CBO	Community-based Organization
CHDC	Child Health and Development Centre
CSO	Civil Society Organization
CPT	Consumer Project on Technology
DANIDA	Danish International Development Agency
DMO	District Medical Officer
FAO	United Nations Food and Agriculture Organization
FIDA	Uganda Women Lawyer's Association
GOU	Government of Uganda
GPPPs	Global Public–Private Partnerships
GTZ	Deutsche Gesellschaft fuer Technische Zusammenarbeit
HIPC	Heavily Indebted Poor Countries
HIV	Human Immunodeficiency Virus
IEC	Information, Education, Communication
IFIs	International Financial Institutions
ILO	International Labour Organization
IMF	International Monetary Fund
IPAA	International Partnership against AIDS in Africa
KAP	Knowledge, Attitude and Practice
LC	Local Council
MAP	World Bank Multi-country HIV/AIDS Project for Africa and the Caribbean
MFPED	Ministry of Finance, Planning and Economic Development (Uganda)
MOH	Ministry of Health
MRC	Medical Research Council (UK)
MSF	Médecins Sans Frontières
NGO	Non-governmental Organization

NRA	National Resistance Army
NRM	National Resistance Movement
ODA	Overseas Development Agency (UK)
PHC	Primary Health Care
RAIN	Rakai AIDS Information Network
RC	Resistance Council
SAPs	Structural Adjustment Policies
SSA	Sub-Saharan Africa
STD	Sexually Transmitted Disease
STI	Sexually Transmitted infection
SYFA	Safeguarding Youth from AIDS
TAC	Treatment Action Campaign (South Africa)
TAG	Treatment Action Group
TASO	The AIDS Support Organization
TB	Tuberculosis
TNCs	Transnational Corporations
TRIPs	Trade-Related Aspects of Intellectual Property Rights
UAC	Uganda AIDS Commission
UNAIDS	Joint United Nations Programme on HIV/AIDS
UNCTAD	United Nations Conference on Trade and Development
UNDP	United Nations Development Programme
UNDCP	United Nations Drug Control Programme
UNFPA	United Nations Fund for Population Activities
UNICEF	United Nations Children's Fund
USAID	United States Agency for International Development
USTR	United States Trade Representative
UVRI	Uganda Virus Research Institute
UWESO	Ugandan Women's Effort to Save the Orphans
WB	World Bank
WBDR	World Bank Development Report
WHO	World Health Organization
WHO/GPA	World Health Organization/Global Programme on AIDS
WID	Women in Development
WTO	World Trade Organization

Introduction: Globalization's Pandemic

Acquired Immune Deficiency Syndrome (AIDS) is a collection of seventy or more conditions, which result from damage caused by a retrovirus to the immune system – the Human Immunodeficiency Virus (HIV). The virus can remain in the body for years before any visible symptoms of the disease appear. The virus chips away at the body's immune system and its host becomes susceptible to other viruses and cancers, until it eventually dies. It is spread from human to human through sex, blood, and from mother to foetus or infant. Extensive spread began in the mid-1970s and AIDS has since become a global pandemic. According to the Joint United Nations Programme on HIV/AIDS (UNAIDS) Epidemic Update of December 2002, 29.4 million out of the 42 million people globally living with HIV infection are in Sub-Saharan Africa (SSA). As of 2000 the continent had buried more than 75 per cent of more than 20 million people who had died of AIDS. In the region, women are infected young, and show a higher prevalence of the disease. And they also shoulder the main burden of the epidemic.

The small trading centre of Lyantonde is located in the southwest of Uganda, on the transnational African highway that begins in Mombasa and runs through Kenya and Uganda to Rwanda. At the height of Uganda's AIDS epidemic, the late 1980s, it was a transient community of approximately 5000 people. Cultivators, mostly women, worked on small plots near their homes. Some women worked in the rest stops and kiosks along the main road, while others sold produce and prepared food in weekly markets in the local area. Traders and long-distance drivers would stop here for rest from their travels. This region had prospered during the height of illegal cross-border trade of the infamous years of Idi Amin's and Milton Obote's rule, from the early 1970s until the mid-1980s. But in 1992 as I travelled through, many of the former hotels and rest stops had been abandoned. HIV prevalence in the trading centres in Rakai peaked at 25 per cent for males and 38 per cent for females in 1989[1]; and in Lyantonde, an estimated 12 per cent of children were orphaned.

At the time, Mrs Muleke lived not far from the trading centre where she cultivated her husband's half-hectare of land. They shared a small mud and wattle house with her mother-in-law, their four children, aged between 7 and 17, and her brother's two orphaned children, aged 1 and 3. Her brother had died of AIDS six months prior, and his wife left the children to find work in Kampala. Mrs Muleke's husband was suffering from AIDS, and her eldest daughter, who had worked as a waitress in the trading centre, had also returned home to die. Her daughter's cash income had helped with the children's school fees, and without this income Mrs Muleke had no choice but to pull the girls out of school. Their labour was now needed in the fields and in caring for the younger children while she tended to her husband and her daughter. Their coffee plot had been lying fallow since her husband became sick, and the other crops were suffering from neglect, but there was still enough of the perennial staple, matooke (green banana), for the family. She had sold the cow to pay for medicines from the pharmacy and the traditional healer, so the children had to go without milk, and it had been a month since they had had meat or fish. The only cash income was from the occasional sale of mats that her mother-in-law produced and sold by the roadside. Mrs Muleke was beginning to feel weak and was losing weight; she feared she too had AIDS. She worried about what would happen to the children when she was gone. Their grandmother was strong, but could not single-handedly care for and support her grandchildren.[2]

In Lyantonde, the formal presence of the AIDS Control Programme (ACP) of the Government of Uganda (GOU) consisted of one woman, whose job was to provide counselling to AIDS sufferers and their families. A research project, directed by a Ugandan physician in partnership with a Canadian researcher, had its office on the main road, and with the community was designing AIDS education strategies. The Rakai AIDS Information Network (RAIN) had recently begun providing counselling and small grants of 500 Uganda shillings (the equivalent of about $50) to HIV-infected people, through its mobile home-care unit that came through the town once a week. The community was struggling to survive through the informal work of grandmothers, who provided what care they could to orphans, of school teachers, who turned down the cash contributions of orphaned children, and through community sharing of local resources. This was in the context of growing impoverishment in Lyantonde related to more general socio-economic decline, a growing debt burden and structural adjustment. Despite a 'rapidly growing economy' in the World Bank's words and the country's adoption of a far-reaching economic reform agenda spearheaded by the International Monetary Fund (IMF) and the World Bank (WB), rural living standards were, and remain, amongst the lowest in the world.

This is a small snapshot of one town in 1992 in Uganda, and of one woman's life. But it is a story that can be repeated in many different parts of SSA today that have been hard hit by AIDS. In Uganda, 10 years later, the prevalence of HIV infection has dropped from an estimated peak of 18.3 per cent in 1992 to 6.5 per cent at the end of 2001,[3] the fall in infections likely the result of a number of factors: the epidemic reaching its saturation point (where so many have died amongst the sexually active population that there is a smaller pool of people still able to acquire the infection); the return of peace and stability in many parts of the country; and Uganda's successful prevention programme, considered a model for the continent.

But infection continues to spread, and the *impacts* of the epidemic – falling *outside* the public health box of the hegemonic analytical model – will continue to be felt for decades to come. Lyantonde reflects the broader geopolitical and economic conditions of the small trading centres and villages that have been hard hit by AIDS. Mrs Muleke's circumstances are typical of the thousands of women who shoulder the major burden of the current AIDS epidemic in Africa south of the Sahara. Her circumstances and options are circumscribed by a harsh global economy in which Uganda is a subordinate player; by political, economic, and legal structures that are a product of Uganda's colonial history and contemporary political economy; by a patriarchal ideology having deep roots in Ugandan sex/gender systems and embodied in contemporary politics and social relations. As with all viruses, HIV can be considered a product of nature and the epidemic, an accident of history. But the evolution of the global epidemic follows patterns that are shaped by human activity and by relations of power that are upheld in the current hegemonic response to HIV.

At a national level, the effects of AIDS on economic growth and production, on the social sectors of health and education, and on human security are beginning to be understood. The complex gender dimensions of HIV spread have also been illuminated, as has the relationship between patterns of HIV spread and long-distance trade, migrant labour, the movement of militaries, war and instability. In fact, the current explanatory frameworks within which HIV/AIDS epidemics in SSA are understood are uncovering important dimensions of the epidemic that have to date been largely marginalized. Yet the institutional response to AIDS in SSA remains focused on the autonomous individual who is to be 'empowered' to protect herself or himself from infection, or cope with imminent death in the absence of treatment.

This book is about AIDS in SSA, with a specific focus on AIDS in Uganda. It is an exploration of the manner in which AIDS has been constructed as a problem of development, and the ways in which AIDS knowledges have evolved and have shaped interventions in the AIDS policy sector. It examines the institutional response to the AIDS epidemic from 1986 to the present, focusing on the activities of a variety of institutions ranging from the World Health Organization (WHO) – the original leaders of global AIDS policy through its Global Programme on AIDS (WHO/GPA), to UNAIDS – the multi-UN agency initiative formed in the mid-1990s, bilateral and multilateral development assistance programmes, foreign and local Civil Society Organizations (CSOs), and the private sector. It necessarily paints a broad brushstroke.

Accompanying the growing AIDS pandemic has been the evolving institutionalization of AIDS expertise. Systems of knowledge about AIDS have been structured by different conceptual frameworks derived from the specific concerns of investigators in various professions and fields. Certain approaches predominate not because they necessarily offer the most comprehensive framework for understanding AIDS, but because of the power and legitimacy of the institutions from which they emerge, and society's faith in their analyses. As Paul Farmer notes,

a critical epistemology of emerging infectious diseases is still in the early stages of development. A key task of this endeavour is to take our existing conceptual frameworks and ask, what is obscured in this way of conceptualising disease? What is brought into relief?[4]

Perhaps most glaringly absent from our knowledge of the global AIDS pandemic is a consideration of how broader economic and social forces contribute to both the shape of emerging epidemics and the policy response. In the case of AIDS in Africa, the politics and ideology of global neoliberalism contribute to the present crisis, and the framework within which the crisis should be addressed; the general acceptance of international competitive rules, liberal economies, the hollowing out of the state, and a belief that market arrangements and the voluntary sector should play a central role in the provision of a minimal social-safety net. Kelly Lee says about global health policy in general:

> Rather than a 'meeting of minds', health policy is being shaped foremost by a broader context of certain value systems, beliefs, aspirations, and so on that seek to maintain a particular world order... debates over how health should be defined are being reframed, from a concern with how to ensure health as a basic human right available to all and collectively provided, to health as a product whose attainment and consumption by individuals should be regulated by the marketplace. This shift is further reflected in the normative criteria, and resultant analytical tools (e.g. burden of disease, cost-effectiveness analysis), which are applied to translate certain values into decisions over, among other things, the allocation of limited health resources.[5]

Neoliberalism is largely consistent with the biomedical construction of AIDS, which reduces the AIDS pandemic to its individual clinical and behavioural dimensions. In effect, what is erased or obscured are the material conditions which allow the virus to thrive, the broader factors that condition access to treatment, and the day-to-day realities of affected households where the tangible impacts are felt. The overwhelming focus on education and clinical management has effectively sidelined other critical dimensions of AIDS – in particular, the gendered crisis of production and reproduction at the local level, a key feature of epidemics in many regions of SSA.

HIV is spread through sex and blood, and biomedical interventions and 'safe-sex' public health campaigns are entirely appropriate. But the distinctive form that the global epidemiology of AIDS has taken is shaped by broader geopolitical and economic forces, which also need to be addressed. Factors shaping epidemics and institutional responses are situated in the broader arena of the global economy and in the offices of the IMF, WB, and World Trade Organization (WTO); in the current pricing and patent protection of drugs to treat HIV infection; in trade liberalization and the promotion of market-driven monoculture; in the privatization of social services including health services; in policies of 'self-reliance' and 'empowerment' which essentially entail that sick bodies fend for themselves. Viral spread and disease response are also conditioned by colonial and post-colonial histories and failed states. My task then is to shift the analysis of AIDS away from an exclusive focus on its clinical and behavioural dimensions, its definition as *only* a health problem and a problem rooted in individual patterns of sexual behaviour, and to analyze AIDS in SSA through the lens of political economy. I should state at the outset that I do not dispute that biomedicine is a successful system for the alleviation of physically or biologically based distress, and I acknowledge biomedicine's central contribution to the under-standing, prevention, and treatment of diseases, AIDS included. But given that biomedicine constructs a hegemonic 'reality', it is important to focus on the good science as well as engage in critique. One effect of biomedicine's hegemony is depoliticizing disease; removing the understanding of disease from its social context and placing it back onto the individual body. The problem rests not with biomedicine per se. It is crucial to understand the relationship between hosts and pathogens. What is troubling is the narrow focus of enquiry into disease – itself related to the power of biomedical discourse and the authority granted to physicians in western societies. Although biomedicine cannot explain more than localized pathological processes, the medical profession and the biomedically trained constitute the majority of top professionals within the major international health policy institutions, WHO/GPA and UNAIDS included.

Global neoliberalism

Globalization in all of its manifestations – social, economic, ideological, cultural, scientific, and technological – has become an object of interrogation within and outside the academy over the past two decades. Volumes have been written about it, so I will not go into great detail here. In its broadest understanding, it refers to processes that have been going on since the early days of conquest and colonization – the inevitable movement towards an integrated world market, the decline of state sovereignty vis-à-vis transnational actors, a convergence of norms on law and human rights, and a homogenization of consumption patterns and cultural expression. If globalization is inevitable, the contemporary form that it has taken is far from 'natural' or inevitable, despite a widespread acceptance that it is. The erosion of real democracy, the kind in which people have an actual say in the establishment of their communities' priorities and the violation of the exercise of the basic human rights of many of the world's inhabitants, is hardly 'natural' or inevitable, nor is the destruction of ecosystems that support human life on the planet. Few can deny that current processes of globalization on the whole have not been beneficial. Heightened prosperity for the minority and rather extreme polarization of wealth have been accompanied by the normalization of extraordinary levels of human suffering.

Contemporary processes of globalization have been managed largely by a (although not exclusively) male, white, affluent elite and have been guided by the specific ideology and set of practices of neoliberalism. Emerging from the leaderships of Thatcher and Reagan in the early 1980s, neoliberalism posits that the rational, isolated individual is the fundamental unit of society, and the market, the natural and just distributor of societies' needs. Humans, by their nature, are competitive utility maximizers, and given the opportunity, their participation in the free market will result in their personal development. Neoliberals view the state as inefficient and often corrupt, whose power encumbers the actions of the market. The role of the neoliberal state is to free markets and maintain the conditions of competition. In the meantime, the reach of the market should be intensified to include all spheres of human activity, including the provision of basic human needs. The specific economic policies of neoliberalism have included the loosening of the mobility of capital and massive tax cuts particularly for the rich and the corporate sector; the privatization of public services such as health, education, utilities, and transportation; an erosion of the rights and protection of workers; and the interpretation of environmental safeguards and legislation as inimical to the free market. Some now speak of the 'post-neoliberal era' where the state is seen as a 'partner' of the market, its new role, to guide and to oversee its workings, and to intervene when it is absolutely necessary.

Globalization in its current guise is not gender neutral. Many scholars and activists have demonstrated how neoliberal restructuring reinforces and exacerbates existing gender inequalities. Early critics illustrated the differential impacts of specific policies of economic restructuring on men and women. The effects of structural adjustment programmes, in particular the rolling back of health, education, and other social services and the elimination of price freezes, on basic goods have intensified women's household labour, as formerly 'public' responsibilities have been rendered 'private' – essentially, shifting responsibility onto the backs of women. Others have examined the processes understood as the 'feminization' of labour – the exponential rise in the number of women workers in casual and flexible sectors of the formal economy, and their increasing numbers in the informal sector – processes that have affected both men and women. In Runyan and Marchand's words, 'the market, the state, and "civil society" (including the "private realm of families/households") are being simultaneously restructured as are the previously assumed boundaries between them'.[6] But as well, the ideology of neoliberalism has served to 'privilege particular agents and sectors over others, such as finance capital over manufacturing, finance ministries over social welfare ministries, the market over the state, the global over the local, consumers over citizens...the latter constructed as "feminized" over the former, which is often depicted as masculine space'.[7] It is difficult not to notice, as they point out, that the new hegemonic masculinity that has emerged privileges the exploits of (white, western, male) global managers over all others. And the linguistics of economics permeates the language of governance – AIDS patients are clients; rural women struggling to hold together fragile communities are potential microentrepreneurs in need only of credit to facilitate their empowerment; cost-effectiveness determines whose life is worth saving. Women's 'private' and caregiving labour is taken as a given – the 'cost-effective' underpinning of market freedom. AIDS policy in Africa is not immune to the neoliberal canon. In the current understanding of AIDS in Africa, the macrostructural features of African economies and societies more broadly are considered mere context for national epidemics, rather than important factors that are shaping the geographic spread of HIV and heightening certain peoples' vulnerability to and risk of infection. The main institutions involved in formulating policy take as a given that states should have a minimal role in the provision of health services, and that the private and voluntary sectors are best equipped to mount the proper response, while others (Oxfam, Save the Children for example) have been critics of the overarching policy framework while operating within it.

The central argument

I suggest that the global institutional response to the AIDS epidemic in SSA was, at first, largely determined by the way that AIDS research and policy proceeded in the west[8] and that despite the attempt to 'globalize' the lens through which epidemics in Africa are understood, the pandemic is still overwhelmingly viewed first and foremost through a biomedical lens, and secondly through a narrow public health lens that focuses on individual sexual behaviour. Within the policy documents on AIDS in Africa, a particular hegemonic understanding of AIDS converges with the ideas and institutional practices of the agencies concerned with the alleviation of poverty in the Third World – shaping the public health response to AIDS. The central focus of AIDS policy is based on the premise that individual sexual-behaviour change brought about by information and education is the main 'weapon' in the fight against AIDS, until the development of a vaccine or cure. In the west, where AIDS is seen largely as a chronic condition, AIDS research and activism has focused overwhelmingly on the drug access problem, while in the Third World, it has been largely taken for granted that widespread treatment is not 'cost-effective', and so prevention takes centre stage, along with individual 'self-help' and empowerment programmes.

The public health response to AIDS in Africa has evolved in the context of massive debt burdens, a crisis in food security, and the failure of states to provide the basic constituents of life, in many instances. In this regard, AIDS policy has evolved in a social and political context that has severely limited policy options. But I think that the problem goes deeper. The hegemonic policy response is unquestioning of the doctrine that the market mechanism should be allowed to direct the fate of human beings. Guaranteeing the fundamental constituents of life takes a back seat to the 'rights' of capital and the establishment of 'free' markets. As Lesley Doyal states, 'it would certainly be foolish to blame "globalization" for the many public health challenges that now face us, but equally, there is clear evidence that restructuring has exacerbated many old problems while also introducing new ones of its own'.[9]

> Health problems themselves are multi-causal and are influenced by factors within both the social and biological realms. A change in the maternal mortality rate, for example, will represent a series of biological events with their own internal logic. However, these deaths will also be related to the social, economic, and cultural configuration of the communities within which they occur, which in turn will be linked in complex ways with aspects of global restructuring.[10]

Grappling with the complex relationship between the biological, the behavioural, and the political economy is less than straightforward. HIV infection is most easily understood as a retrovirus spread through bodily fluids. This study is one modest attempt to sharpen the lens through which disease and globalization is understood – as a complex articulation of the biological, the behavioural, and the political economy. It also serves as an indictment of neoliberalism's underlying economic and moral doctrine, which continues to justify the denial of people's access to the most basic level of subsistence and care.

The outline of this book

The first three chapters focus on SSA as a whole, and are meant to illuminate the broad contours of the political economy of HIV/AIDS on the sub-continent. The next two chapters focus on one country – Uganda – as a means of giving concrete expression to some of the general ideas developed earlier in the book. The first chapter, 'AIDS Knowledges and the Africa's Pandemic', focuses on how SSA is understood in the global AIDS pandemic. It provides a brief historical sketch of the competing knowledge systems of AIDS – the predominant understandings that have informed the global policy response, their social conditions, and institutional contexts. I begin with an account of AIDS and medical science, and the social and political construction of AIDS in the western world. Research on HIV/AIDS has been dominated by the medical sciences, the main informants of the public health response in the west, where most research is carried out, and in the Third World where National AIDS Programmes have largely been the recipients of the wisdom of western-based institutions. As well, competing social and moral understandings have shaped AIDS policy, as have advocacy movements, both local and global. In the past decade, the understanding of AIDS in SSA has evolved from a principally biomedical/behavioural paradigm to a broader understanding that views AIDS as a broader problem of development with multiple effects.

How that more nuanced, multidimensional understanding has conditioned the policy response is the subject of Chapter 2, 'Africa in the Global Institutional Response'. It focuses on the politics of the evolution of the international policy response, from the formation of the WHO/GPA to the joint UN initiative of UNAIDS and the 'global multi-sectoral strategy'. I discuss the ways in which various sectors – governments, bilateral and multilateral institutions, non-governmental organizations (NGOs) and the voluntary sector, the private sector and charitable foundations, and 'civil society' – have been brought into the implementation of the response on the ground. A separate chapter is devoted to the issue of access to life-saving drugs; Chapter 3, 'The Other "War on Drugs"', discusses how SSA has been situated in the politics of Antiretroviral (ARV) therapy and vaccine development. My main focus is on developments since the formation of the WTO and the expansion of international trade law into the sphere of pharmaceutical research and development as codified in Trade-Related Aspects of Intellectual Property Rights (TRIPS), and the political activism surrounding the issue of access to life-saving drugs.

The next two chapters focus specifically on Uganda, the country where it is widely believed that HIV originated, the first country in SSA to respond, and today considered the 'African Success Story' for halting the epidemic in its tracks. Chapter 4, 'Why Africa? Uganda's Epidemic in Historical Perspective', is an implicit challenge to the main assumptions underlying current AIDS control and prevention strategies that view the disease through a biomedical and behavioural lens, problematizing the dominant view of 'culture' that underlies many current AIDS prevention campaigns on the continent where culture is understood as a separate realm of ideas and values intrinsic to particular ethnic groupings that prevent them from practicing safe sex. The social/moral orders influencing sexual relations are considered in relation to broader historical processes. The chapter explores the foundations of the current political economy and the socio-cultural context of AIDS in Uganda. It discusses Uganda's pre-independence history not only to highlight the general political context of today's institutional response to the epidemic, but also to mark the features of the region's economic development and political and social history that help to explain the contemporary spread of HIV. The transformation of gender and sexual relations and previous epidemics of Sexually Transmitted Diseases (STDs) in the Great Lakes region is considered in the context of the disruptions to kin-corporate societies resulting from colonial social and economic policy and the changes in systems of governance imposed by the colonial state. I then address the nature of the post-colonial Ugandan state and political economy, providing the context for understanding patterns of HIV spread in Uganda, as well as the institutional response.

Chapter 5, 'The Uganda "Success Story"', examines the institutional response to the epidemic in Uganda from 1986 to the present. The policy response is considered in a number of respects: the colonial and immediate post-colonial legacy; the vision of AIDS control embodied in the central donor institutions; and the adoption of a neoliberal economic agenda and Structural Adjustment Policies (SAPs), which undermined the re-establishment of basic health services throughout the country and put severe constraints on the effectiveness of interventions. The objective is to illuminate how government policy and development assistance in the AIDS sector has been conditioned, not only by a particular hegemonic understanding of HIV/AIDS in Africa which focuses principally on the individual and the disease as units of analysis, but also by the context within which the various agencies have, and continue, to operate. The analysis situates HIV/AIDS policy in the light of the structural contradictions of the Ugandan state and the socio-economic conditions that circumscribe the room for manoeuvre of institutions, both large and small.

The Conclusion, 'AIDS, Human Rights, and Global Inequality', weaves together the various threads of the analysis to argue for a strengthened human rights perspective on AIDS. As with all viruses, HIV can be considered a product of nature, and the epidemic, an accident of history. But the evolution of the AIDS pandemic follows patterns that are shaped by human activity *and* by relations of power that are upheld in the current hegemonic response to AIDS; underpinning power in the current global order is an understanding of 'rights' not as claims to real developmental needs.

A note on method

The empirical research of this book had its beginnings in the summer of 1989 when I was carrying out interviews with traditional healers in the Kampala area on the relationship between traditional therapies and the formal health care system. My research did not specifically focus on HIV/AIDS, but 'slim', as it was called then, was raised repeatedly in the course of my research. Billboards and bumper stickers were advising people to 'love carefully' and to 'zero graze', and The AIDS Support Organization (TASO), had a visible presence in Kampala. The AIDS sector in Uganda was one of the fastest growing, and the urgency of the problem and the seemingly quick mobilization of the Ugandan government to respond piqued my interest.

I returned to Uganda in 1992 to carry out doctoral research, and the book draws from this research. The first two months were spent at the Makerere University Library, the Mengo Hospital Archives, the Medical Library of Mulago Hospital, the Makerere Institute of Social Research and Centre for Basic Research in Kampala, and the Government Archives in Entebbe. Research focused on the evolution of the migrant labour system during the colonial period, the history of the treatment of STDs in Uganda, gender relations and the law, and general historical and contemporary political economy. By this time, my research agenda had been approved by the Uganda AIDS Commission (UAC) and the National Council of Science and Technology and I received a formal research permit. The next months focused on research into the institutional analysis, which included analyzing policy and project documents from the main organizations involved in AIDS control in Uganda, interviewing their representatives (see Appendix), as well as visiting hard-hit communities and key AIDS-related projects. The analysis also draws from primary research carried out in Uganda by other researchers, both academic and policy oriented. In-depth discussions with men and women from the districts of Rakai, Masaka, Kampala, and Jinja were carried out throughout the course of the research – case studies of how the epidemic had affected the daily lives of ordinary men and women. I also draw on research that I collected from a 400-household survey on general health, socio-economic conditions, rural–urban population movements, and gender relations in the town of Jinja. The survey, conducted with Makerere sociologist Arnest Wabwire, was part of an urban study conducted with the Jinja Municipal Council and funded by the Canadian International Development Agency. In 1996, Gonzaaga Busuulwu, my research assistant from the Child Health and Development Centre (CHDC) at Mulago Hospital, sent me updated epidemiological and AIDS surveillance reports from the ACP, recent publications of the UAC, United Nations Childrens Fund (UNICEF), CARE, and some key research reports to update some of the demographic and epidemiological data. I also draw from the vast body of scholarship that has been produced since that time, both scholarly and policy oriented.

Since the early 1990s, the production of knowledge related to HIV/AIDS in SSA has increased exponentially – the bibliography on which this book is based constitutes a small fraction of the research produced over the past decade. What follows represents one account of 'globalization's pandemic'; my hope is that it can contribute in more than just a theoretical way to how we understand the relationship between globalization and disease spread, and open up new pathways to understand the complex gender dynamics underpinning human health and the exercise of basic human rights.

Notes

1. Tony Barnett and Piers Blaikie, *AIDS in Africa: Its Present and Future Impact* (London: Bellhaven Press, 1992) 32.
2. Some details of Mrs Muleke's story, as well as her name, have been changed.
3. GOU Ministry of Health, based on data from selected antenatal sentinel sites (http://health.go.ug/hiv).
4. Paul Farmer, *Infections and Inequalities: The Modern Plagues* (Berkeley: University of California Press, 2001) 40.
5. Kelley Lee, Kent Buse, and Suzanne Fustukian, eds, *Health Policy in a Globalizing World* (Cambridge: Cambridge University Press, 2002) 10.
6. Marianne H. Marchand and Anne Sisson Runyan, eds, *Gender and Global Restructuring: Sightings, Sites and Resistances* (London: Routledge, 2000) 226.
7. Marchand and Runyan, 13.

8. By 'west' I am referring to the industrialized capitalist countries of North America and Western Europe. Most AIDS research is carried out in the US, France, Germany, and Canada.
9. Lesley Doyal, 'Putting Gender into Health and Globalization Debates: New Perspectives and Old Challenges', *Third World Quarterly* 23 (2002): 237.
10. Doyal, 235.

1

AIDS Knowledges and Africa's Pandemic

> In the emerging literature on emerging infectious diseases, some questions are posed while others are not. A subtle and flexible understanding of emerging infections would be grounded in critical and reflexive study of how our knowledge develops. Units of analysis and key terms would be scrutinized and regularly redefined. These processes would include regular rethinking not only of methodologies and study design but also of the validity of causal inference, and they would allow reflection on the limits of human knowledge.
>
> Paul Farmer, *Infections and Inequalities:*
> *The Modern Plagues*

On one end of the spectrum of AIDS knowledges, AIDS is a microbe, understood through the tools of modern virology, immunology, and molecular biology; in the middle of the spectrum, it is a disease spread largely through culturally defined patterns of sexual behaviour; and on the other end, a virus whose prevalence and impact vary according to a country's socio-economic and political status and position within the global political economy. Shaping the policy response to the global pandemic are principally the first two understandings, reflecting both the power of biomedical and public health approaches to disease in general, and the boundaries of knowledge set by disciplinary enquiry. What is just beginning to emerge is an understanding of AIDS, which situates its manifestation in relation to gendered global, regional, and local distributions of power and resources, accounts for variations on the basis of local specificities, and questions biological individualism without rejecting biology.

The knowledge that underpins the policy approaches to AIDS, far from being objective and value-free, constructs the epidemic in certain ways. The understanding of AIDS has been produced in the social world, and the use and the results of that knowledge are political. Some questions are asked, while others are ignored. Knowledge is partial and often reflects the vested interests of the actors involved. Who decides on the priorities assigned for AIDS research? How are those priorities determined? What follows provides just a sketch of the evolution of how African AIDS has been understood within the global pandemic. I begin with a brief account of AIDS and medical science in the 'western' world, given that research on AIDS has been dominated by the medical sciences, the main informants of the public health response both in the west where most research is carried out and in the 'Third World' where National AIDS programmes have largely been the recipients of the wisdom of western-based institutions. I then move on to discuss the competing social and moral understandings that have shaped the direction of western AIDS policy, and AIDS-specific advocacy movements, particularly those organized by gay men who initially were the main focus of research and public health campaigns. The discussion then moves to consider how Africa has been understood in the global pandemic. The understanding of AIDS in Africa lies in a complex mix of biomedicine, behaviourism, a wider moral and political agenda, and the development, security, and human rights discourses of the past decades.

The hegemony of biomedicine

> In the paradigm of clinical medicine...diseases are biological, universal, and ultimately transcend social and cultural context.[1]

Western societies are deeply committed to biomedicine as the main institution for both producing knowledge about human disease and responding to it. As an institution, it has authority over the many other systems of medicine that are practiced; as Paul Starr contends, no other system has systematically assembled a body of knowledge expressed so fully in texts, refereed journal articles, and clinical studies.

Its power resides in a vast system of hospitals, clinics, research institutes, pharmaceutical and insurance companies, and other organizations; and its authority rests on its view of medical reality through definitions of disease and health which are reproduced from one generation to the next.[2] Endlessly repeated within a narrow context of meaning, biomedicine's truths are rarely scrutinized as partial. Indeed, when we are sick, we want to understand what is wrong with us, and we want treatment to make us better. But we tend to ask less frequently why we get sick in the first place.

Biomedicine was not always so powerful. Paul Starr's history of American medicine suggests that originally, public health had closer affiliations with engineering than with medicine, with the early efforts of sanitarians directed at 'cleansing' the environment. The evolution of the field of bacteriology in the late 1800s led to a more precise conception of the modes of transmission of particular pathogens, shifting focus from the environment to the human carriers of disease. But Starr also depicts the very notion of public health as politically subversive and an invitation to conflict, its history throughout the nineteenth and twentieth centuries being a tug of war with private practitioners over the limits of its mandate. Public health authorities met opposition from business and commerce, who saw the enactment of public health legislation as 'municipal socialism' and unfair competition with private business. At the end of the nineteenth century, both the moral and the economic boundaries of public health were contested as public health agencies intruded into the activities that the medical profession believed to be rightly its own.[3] Leslie Doyal contends that in the early nineteenth century, public health measures in fact aided in the consolidation of biomedicine's authority, by helping to bring major epidemic illnesses under control. Better living and working conditions, improved hygiene, sanitation, and nutrition were overlooked by a medical profession that paid less attention to 'the societies within which bodies lived their lives'.[4] Health policy in the industrialized world has overwhelmingly emphasized after-the-event curative medical intervention and has paid little attention to broadly based measures to prevent people from getting sick in the first place. Public health specialists have tended to share the underlying assumptions of biomedicine to the extent that public health campaigns are largely focused on individual-behaviour modification through lifestyle changes. According to Barnett and Whiteside,

Neither public health nor clinical medicine pays sufficient attention to what does improve health – escaping from poverty, access to good food, clean water, sanitation, shelter, education, and preventative care. Clinical medicine has marginal effects on people's long term health.[5]

But the problem is not simply that clinical medicine fails to pay sufficient attention, but that it is difficult for our highly individualistic societies to *see* the link between the broader organization of societies, the distribution of wealth and power, and human health. Unfettered growth and trade, understood as 'freedom', overrides other values. Today, it is not necessarily that health practitioners do not see the obvious – many, in fact, do. The mandate of biomedical doctors is to treat disease in the individual body. In relatively affluent parts of the world, where the basic constituents of health are taken for granted by most people, clinical and high-tech medicine has much to offer. In contexts where disease burden largely stems from malnutrition, pesticide poisoning, unemployment, harsh working conditions, and structural violence, its limitations are obvious. Today, biomedicine is largely a commodity in the free market to be purchased by those who can pay, or to be accessed by the increasingly fewer number who have private or public insurance, most of who live in the west. Drugs are not considered public goods, essential to health and are not distributed based on need, but are a multibillion dollar industry, and research on drugs is overwhelmingly focused on profitable diseases. Africa constitutes a mere one per cent of the global pharmaceutical market, while North America, Western Europe, and Japan together constitute 80 per cent.[6] According to the WHO, 25–66 per cent of health spending in low-income countries is on pharmaceuticals, where in most, they constitute the largest household expenditure among the poor. Fifty to ninety per cent pay out of their pockets and the expense of family illness is a major cause of household impoverishment. The proliferation of profit-making firms in medical services and the consolidation of a narrow biomedical frame for understanding human health are global phenomenons.

AIDS emerged at the time of neoliberalism's global consolidation. The current understanding of AIDS in Africa is largely compatible with neoliberalism to the extent that the focus is on the isolated individual, abstracted from broader social relations. However, over the past two decades, the biomedical and behavioural model has been broadened and deepened, and an evolving understanding of how the absence of the basic constituents of health has shaped pathogenesis, risk behaviour, and access to treatment and care is beginning to emerge.

The emergence of a new epidemic

According to Gerald Oppenheimer, competing sub-fields of medical research on AIDS have been virology, immunology, and epidemiology, with epidemiology straddling the line between the medical and social science. Epidemiologists obtained institutional control over AIDS research early on in the epidemic.

> Faced with a disease of unknown origin, epidemiologists and their collaborators constructed, over time, hypothetical models to explain the disorder in order to contain it. Prior to the isolation of a putative causal agent, HIV, epidemiologists played a central role in defining the new syndrome, first developing a 'lifestyle' model, and later, a model based on hepatitis B. Although later supplanted by their position by virologists and other bench scientists working in laboratories, epidemiologists have continued to define important dimensions of the disorder and to raise disquieting questions. Specifically, they were concerned with defining the natural history of HIV infection, the extent to which it had spread within population groups, and the factors that affected rates of disease – factors beyond the virus itself.[7]

Epidemiology explains broad patterns of disease seeking to 'measure and analyze the occurrence and distribution of diseases and other health-related conditions, acting as both a sentinel who warns of shifts in disease patterns and as a scout who seizes on such shifts to discover their aetiology'.[8] As Nancy Krieger explains, a complex web of numerous interconnected risk and protective factors explains broad population patterns of health and disease. Through disease surveillance, epidemiologists discern changes in disease distribution within particular populations on the basis of which they formulate hypotheses concerning the relation between the disease and the variables that may affect its natural history and clinical course – the objective to isolate the causal variables of the disease. Contemporary epidemiology incorporates environmental factors into its understanding of the disease, but the tendency has been to interpret them in a narrow and selective frame, emphasizing variables that can be linked very directly to the disease in question. Indeed, some epidemiologists have been critical of the acceptance of purely biomedical explanations of the disease and limited models of aetiology within epidemiology.

In the early days of the AIDS epidemic, initial research was driven by the hypothesis that the new syndrome was a consequence of promiscuity and drug abuse. When the new disease was first detected in North America, its first sufferers were a small number of gay men. The fact that they were all young male homosexuals suggested to epidemiologists a link between 'homosexual lifestyle' and immune dysfunction. The 'immune overload' hypothesis focused on such factors as persistent STD infection, numerous sex partners, attendance at bathhouses, a history of syphilis, and exposure to faeces during sex. The first informal label attached to the new disease reflected this; it was known as Gay-related Immune Deficiency (GRID) until similar opportunistic infections began to appear outside the gay community. According to Steven Epstein, the new syndrome was framed as a gay man's disease to the point where 'medical practitioners and researchers sometimes resisted the idea that it might appear elsewhere, and those who proposed that the epidemic could affect other people risked being discredited within the scientific community'.[9] The understanding of AIDS as a disease 'caused' by 'rampant promiscuity' never went away – AIDS from the beginning signified a disease confined to particular risk groups and social locations.

By 1983, there was mounting evidence of similar opportunistic infections occurring in people around the world, and in the US rising numbers of infections outside the 'gay community'. Added to the 'risk group' of homosexual men were Haitians, heroin addicts, and haemophiliacs, this latter group portrayed in the popular media as the 'innocent victims' of the emerging epidemic. After virologists at the Pasteur Institute in Paris and the National Cancer Institute in the US concurrently isolated a virus, in 1984, believed to be the cause of the new disease, the understanding of the syndrome shifted from a purely 'lifestyle' based disease to one based on transmissible agent spread through blood, this model supporting the introduction of public health measures.[10] In the absence of a cure or vaccine, behavioural changes were crucial to stemming the tide of infection. The solution was relatively simple – avoid sharing body fluids. Given the high concentration of infection among gay men in North America and the fact that they mobilized early on in the epidemic, women remained invisible in AIDS research, despite rising levels of infection in women in other parts of the world. In Africa, roughly equal numbers of men and women were infected with HIV. In the US, many of the women who were becoming infected were poor blacks, Latinas, and intravenous drug users, living on the margins of society and the main targets of Ronald Reagan's cuts in federal spending on social services. Paul Farmer poses the question: why did many continue to think of AIDS as a men's disease?

> One explanation is that the majority of women with AIDS had been robbed of their voices long before HIV appeared to further complicate their lives. In settings of entrenched elitism, they have been poor. In settings of entrenched racism, they have been women of colour. In settings of entrenched sexism, they have been, of course, women.[11]

The isolation of a virus held out the promise of clinical management of the new syndrome. The claim that HIV was the etiological agent in AIDS was the guiding assumption behind billion-dollar programmes for the HIV-antibody testing, antiviral drug development and treatment, and vaccine research around the world.[12] By 1986, the view that HIV was the cause of AIDS was hegemonic, but Epstein describes the controversy that never went away and extended across a range of scientific disciplines. Some of the questions that were raised, and that continue to be raised, focused on whether HIV was indeed the causal agent, whether it was the sole cause of AIDS or whether cofactors needed to be present; other controversies have centred on broader issues or questions about the politics of treatment such as whether the drugs being developed and prescribed at high prices were poisonous in themselves.

> The actors in this drama are as varied as the interests that motivate them and the values that animate them – the researchers hoping to hit on breakthroughs in the basic or applied sciences of AIDS research; the pharmaceutical and biotechnology companies whose stock values might fluctuate by millions of dollars, depending on

the latest reports about the successes or failures of their products; the medical professionals who must translate inconclusive and contradictory research into workable, day-to-day clinical judgments; the regulatory agencies and advisory bodies that serve as 'gate-keepers', ruling on the safety and efficacy of new therapies; the patients who consume the drugs and populate the clinical trials; the reporters and journalists who interpret scientific findings to various segments of the public, and of course, the activists who police the whole process and offer their own interpretations of the methods and the outcomes.[13]

The activists in this regard largely consisted of gay men, who became instrumental in challenging the science as well as the public policy of AIDS. Despite the stigmatized status of gays in North America and Europe, relatively affluent members of the community in particular were able to play an active role in challenging and shaping the response to the epidemic. As Epstein explains, white, middle-class men dominated gay communities – people with influence in society and with an array of social, cultural, and political resources.[14] 'AIDS became a "gay disease" primarily because clinicians, epidemiologists, and reporters perceived it through that filter, but secondarily because gay communities were obliged to make it their own.'[15] Unlike other 'risk groups' (poor women and intravenous drug users, for example), there was a gay community based on a shared identity, with financial resources to mount an active campaign. The discourse of AIDS activism reflected a conflict between traditional public health approaches such as contact tracing and imposing restrictions on the rights of the HIV infected, and pressure to respect individual human rights and civil liberties – defined as the rights to privacy, bodily autonomy, and freedom from discrimination. In Epstein's words, 'AIDS activists sought to challenge the ideological linkages between sex and death and put forward sex-positive programs of AIDS prevention that assert the right to sexual pleasure and sexual freedom.'[16] Gay-community organization represented a comparatively successful campaign at a time when few CSOs were able to make claims on the state.

The understanding of AIDS in the West gradually shifted in the mid-to late 1980s, from one of 'fatal' to 'chronic' disease. Drug research and development began to move at a fast pace, but with much more interest on the part of the pharmaceutical industry in developing treatments to keep the virus at bay, rather than in discovering an unprofitable vaccine. Resources were skewed to developing a cure and highly effective ARV therapy with its huge profits and cost of $10,000–30,000 a year for the drugs alone. Drugs research, some of it conducted in Africa under dubious ethical standards, has so far proven largely irrelevant to 90 per cent of the world's HIV-infected population. Furthermore, biomedical research that might have benefited women, such as the development of female-controlled barrier methods and topical microbicides, was also slow to develop.

But also important in shaping the public health response to AIDS in the west was the turn toward neoliberal economics, and its accompanying moral and political agenda. The AIDS pandemic emerged in conjunction with the increasing withdrawal of the state from the social sectors, privatization, and the opening up of economies to global market forces. The two competing discourses that gave AIDS its cultural meaning in the US were both compatible with the neoliberal political agenda: the discourse of the 'moral majority' on the one hand and the counterdiscourse of civil libertarianism on the other. Within the evangelical right wing, AIDS became a major issue through which to challenge the evolving acceptance of sexualities and family forms brought about by gay rights and feminist movements. For the evangelical right wing, AIDS was seen as a punishment from God for those who deviated from the patriarchal, monogamous, nuclear family. Says Simon Watney, prominent gay activist and cultural critic of US and British AIDS policy:

> What AIDS commentary does is to elide the virus and its presenting symptoms with the dominant cultural meanings of those constituencies in which it emerged – black Africans, injecting drug users, prostitutes, and of course, gay men. In this manner, 'the social' is ever more narrowly confined with familial definitions and values, with the family being scrutinized ever more closely for physical symptoms of moral dissent.[17]

Resistance of the gay community was characterized by an explicit discourse of individual rights. Social movement politics in the US had a not-insignificant effect on the global movement. Agencies like the Clarence Higgins Trust in Britain and the Gay Men's Health Crisis in New York became international models of grassroots AIDS organizing.

In an in-depth international survey of the first AIDS service organizations conducted by the Global AIDS Policy Commission in 1992, it was found that over half had been founded by a group of predominantly gay men, usually self-identified as white and middle class. States Jeff O'Malley, author of the report, 'The contribution of gay men and lesbians to creating an ASO movement is most notable in the industrialized countries, but was also relevant to the creation of AIDS Service Organizations (ASOs) in the developing world, particularly in Latin America and Southeast Asia, and even, in discrete fashion, in at least three sub-Saharan African countries.'[18] Despite its relative successes, the application of the western model of AIDS organizing to Africa was not unambiguous. As this model was imported to African countries, so too was the discourse of AIDS and human rights, which initially focused almost exclusively on individual rights to bodily autonomy, privacy, and freedom from stigma and discrimination.[19] Few would dispute the importance of antidiscriminatory measures. But the almost exclusive focus on stigma and discrimination arose from a conception of human rights that was both liberal and androcentric in that it assumed a level of bodily autonomy that most people, particularly women, did not have – what Scheper-Hughes describes as sexual citizenship:

> a broad constellation of individual, medical, social, and legal rights designed to protect bodily autonomy, bodily integrity, reproductive freedom, and sexual equity. Sexual citizenship implies, among other things, the ability to negotiate the kind of sex one wants, freedom from rape and other forms of non-consensual or coercive sex, and freedom from forced reproduction and coerced abortion.[20]

Absent at the time from the discourse on AIDS and human rights was an understanding of how the denial of the exercise of basic rights to bodily autonomy and basic needs shaped both the risk of infection and the ability to cope with its multiple impacts. Farmer describes the subtle discrimination against poor, HIV-positive single mothers in the US who were denied access to clinical trials on the basis of their non-compliance; contributing to their non-compliance were the daily struggles of maintaining a household and caring for children against all odds such as not having the bus fare or the childcare to attend appointments, and of being in the position of caring for others without support while needing care oneself.[21] In the highly individualistic culture of the US, AIDS sufferers living on the margins remained the most stigmatized – poor women in particular, whose stigmatization was linked to the broader workings of social and gender inequality. But it was a discourse compatible with a policy response whose main elements were prevention through educational campaigns and treatment for those who could afford to pay.

Understanding African AIDS

In the course of two decades, Africa moved from being marginal to the AIDS epidemic to being the 'global epicentre', leading to a dramatic influx of international collaboration for medical and social research on virology, immunology, epidemiology, and pathogenesis, and for an endless stream of knowledge production. A significant difference between the 'western' epidemic and emerging epidemics in the 'Third World' was the roughly equal numbers of males and females infected in the Third World. In Africa, heterosexual transmission was estimated to account for between 80 and 90 per cent of all cases, the other 20 per cent, a combination of perinatal transmission and infections through contaminated blood. The geographic distribution of AIDS in Africa has been far from uniform, with the first infections clustered in the Rakai District of Uganda. By 1988, the WHO was collecting case data from the majority of countries in Africa, showing a concentration of infection in the Great Lakes region of Uganda, Tanzania, Congo, Burundi, Kenya, Rwanda, Zambia, and Zaire. Under 10,000 cases were reported at this time, but at least one case had been reported in 41 countries.[22]

The main question guiding research on AIDS in Africa was: what is distinct about the heterosexual spread of HIV in African countries? Scientists initially looked to parallels with the western experience to guide research on the epidemiology of AIDS. Sexual behaviour became the main focus of research. According to Brooke Grundfest Schoepf, biological frameworks mixed with certain assumptions about African sexuality initially determined the questions asked, and medical doctors, as members of the dominant discipline controlling major funding, established the initial terms of enquiry.[23] Researchers from other disciplines – public health specialists, anthropologists, and economists – also contributed insights into that which could not be explained by the clinically trained alone.

One assumption guiding scientific research was that the high levels of HIV infection in Africa pointed to the continent as the origin of the virus. HIV in humans was hypothesized to be a simian immuno-deficiency virus that had mutated once a crossover from an animal to a human carrier had occurred, most likely from the African green monkey. The movement of viruses from animals to humans is fairly common, as is the study of the origin of viruses, which often yields crucial information for the management of viral epidemics. The Green monkey cross-over hypothesis was inherently neutral, regardless of its scientific plausibility. But the western portrayal of AIDS in Africa in the media as a virus infecting Africans through the eating of uncooked monkey meat and then spreading like wildfire because of rampant promiscuity and polygamy ignited a well-justified backlash in some African communities and added fuel to the fire of conspiracy theories that AIDS was a form of biological warfare from the west – a strategy to depopulate the continent.

In the early research on the transmission of AIDS in Africa, the rapid spread of HIV was seen as a consequence of factors such as traditional ritual practices; young at age during the first sexual activity, high levels of premarital sex, high levels of extramarital sexual relations, polygamy, wife-sharing, widow inheritance, funeral rights, scarification, and circumcision using dirty instruments.[24] Other practices such as anal intercourse and 'dry sex' – the insertion of leaves and powders into the vagina which resulted in injury to soft tissue and augmented viral transmission in women – also received some attention in early research.[25] Particular risk groups set apart from the general population were young single women, who worked in bars as prostitutes, and long-distance lorry drivers. Factors viewed to be contributing to high levels of promiscuity were migration, alcohol consumption, 'poverty', and the breakdown of traditional moral codes with increased urban-ization and modernization. 'Poor knowledge' and reluctance to use condoms were also factors. To a certain degree, the emerging under-standing of the sexual behaviour of Africans was marked by a debate about whether Africans were or were not promiscuous, the debate itself reflecting a particular standard of morality and the notion that sexual fidelity is the natural order.[26] The overwhelming focus on certain risk groups led to victim-blaming and repressive measures, particularly of commercial sex workers, who were singled out initially as one of the main 'vectors of transmission'. While 'prostitutes' were targeted as a problem, elite urban men were initially exempt from consideration, despite the fact that many were the ones paying for sexual services.

It was the role of epidemiologists and anthropologists to explain the specific behavioural patterns underlying the spread of HIV among the heterosexual population in Africa. Although there is great diversity in the conceptual approaches adopted by various researchers, the majority of studies originally aligned with ACPs focused on the rational, isolated individual as the unit of analysis – their goal to 'uncover the facts' about high-risk sexual behaviour. Survey research was conducted among designated 'high-risk' groups. In countries like Zaire, Tanzania, and Uganda, popular cohorts were prostitutes, pregnant women, long-distance lorry drivers, and patients at STD clinics. KAP surveys, KAP the abbreviation for 'knowledge, attitude, practice', were a popular methodological instrument for obtaining information on sexual 'risk behaviours' related to HIV spread, on the basis of which educational interventions would be formulated. The Population Council in New York originally developed KAP questionnaires in the early 1960s.[27] Underpinning KAP surveys is a specific atomistic model of culture; culture is understood as the sum of individual knowledge and behaviours, and can be reduced to its component parts. The information gathered through a KAP study, once codified by a qualified social scientist, would then become the basis for behavioural change interventions. According to Barnett and Whiteside, 'the resulting programmes were firmly based on the tradition of individual psychology and on two main theories: the Health Belief Model and the Theory of Reasoned Action and Planned Behaviour'. Both theories assume ontological monism – humans are rational actors, who when presented with proper knowledge and a stimulus will modify their actions.

Certainly in an epidemic, it is important to understand how the virus is spread – the focus on sexual behaviour was justified. Some researchers, however, pointed to the embedded and sometimes blatant racism surfacing in scientific and popular accounts of sexual behaviour, as well as the limitations of research that viewed sexual behaviour as private acts distinct from other social forces and relations. Grundfest Schoepf, for example, leader of a collaborative action-research team studying AIDS in Zaire in the latter half of 1990, described the discussion of sexual behaviour in Africa as 'surrounded by value-laden assumptions and charged with political implications...rooted in

Western constructions of Africans as "primitives" whose "unfettered sexuality" is envied, coveted and feared'.[28] Schoepf and others pointed to the problems with certain approaches to research that failed to consider the social and economic conditions that gave rise to certain risk behaviours – conditions rooted in colonial histories and contemporary political economies.

Another area of research existing on the margins was a consideration of the potential biological cofactors that rendered people vulnerable to infection. The notion that AIDS was spread because of 'rampant promiscuity' was so entrenched that other hypotheses for the efficient spread of the virus on the African continent received little consideration. Stillwaggon points out that biomedical factors that promote HIV infection, particularly among very poor people, have been overlooked because of the narrow framing of policy in behavioural terms which made more sense in the US and Europe.[29] By the early 1990s, it was established that chronic and untreated STDs – present in large numbers in certain regions – presented an up to eight times greater risk of transmission and, in turn, impaired immunity. Stillwaggon provides substantial evidence that malnutrition and parasitosis compromise the function of the immune system, rendering people more susceptible to HIV as well as other infectious diseases. These biological conditions, nested in poverty and an absence of basic health care services, were eclipsed by the almost exclusive focus on sexual behaviour.

A deepening of the knowledge base

But the focus on sexual behaviour underwent a subtle shift as time went on, given that campaigns seemed to be having a limited impact on HIV spread. Helen Epstein comments on the effectiveness of prevention programmes in Uganda pointing to the emergence of two schools of thought: 'Either people's beliefs about condoms, fertility, and disease prevent them from practicing safe sex or they are constrained by the larger social conditions in their lives, such as poverty and unemployment, that result in a kind of resignation, a feeling that HIV is inevitable, and beyond one's power to prevent.'[30] Sexual behaviour was increasingly understood in the broader context of civil war and instability, single-gender labour migration and the separation of household members, and gender relations, particularly women's economic dependence on men and the cultural imperative to have children. Stated elegantly by Dominique Frommel,

> The research done by UNAIDS, coupled with the experience of the WHO and UNICEF in the field of human reproduction, will undoubtedly reveal how diverse sexuality is, but can all this information pinpoint what is needed to motivate men and women who have been warned about HIV to change their behaviour and sexual practices? Or will it just lead to pointless arguments that conceal the scale of the social and economic factors which impede changes in sexual behaviour?[31]

In the early 1990s, 'Women and AIDS' became a focus within AIDS research, the Women and Development directorates of many bilateral and multilateral institutions developing a space for themselves (albeit a small and separate one) among the medical doctors and public health specialists. At this time, there was a growing understanding that women were more at risk – surveillance data indicated that women were becoming infected younger, and female infections began to outstrip males in some regions. Apart from research on women's specific biological vulnerability, studies began to appear on the social, economic, and legal status of women, and its relationship to risk of infection. Survey and ethnographic research pointed to women's lack of decision-making power in sexual relationships (did they have the power in their relationships to insist on condom use?) and the difficulty of practicing 'safe sex' in a context where women's self-worth was measured largely by their capacity to reproduce, and where children provided some measure of security in an unstable economic environment. Research also pointed to the particular problems of AIDS widows who would find themselves destitute when they lost rights to children and property upon the death of their husbands, as well as the limited income-earning options of impoverished women who were selling sexual services.

Research carried out in rural and peri-urban areas of Uganda, Zimbabwe, and Zaire on women's risk of contracting infection demonstrated that risk was shaped by a number of historical factors; women's tenuous legal position regarding property and inheritance, their exclusion from the cash economy, as well as the intransigence of an ideology of men's ownership of women's productive and reproductive labour. Women were largely excluded from the economic security of owning land and from cash economies which were largely under male control. Focusing on the micropolitics of survival in the Rakai District of Uganda, Barnett and Blaikie described the ways in which some women survived through different types of relationships with men, such as providing a range of domestic services, preparing food and brewing beer, and providing lodging as well as sex and companionship.[32] Similar observations were made regarding sexual relations in Zimbabwe by Bassett and Mhloyi[33] and by Grundfest Schoepf with reference to Kinshasa, Zaire:

> Long distance traders are likely to have several wives or women whom they live in relatively stable unions in towns along their routes. Wives and children provide the trader with an identity as a responsible adult with a reason for being in the town. Their houses shelter the husband's activities from the prying eyes that follow hotel guests and also provide secure storage of goods. Wives make trading contacts and also obtain permits using their local kinship and patron–client networks. They also may trade on their own account with goods or capital supplied by the visiting husbands. Some of these wives are monogamous; others have two or more husbands. As economic conditions continue to worsen, sexual strategies which maximize returns become increasingly important. While no statistics exist, our observations indicate that multiple partner unions, particularly those involving various forms of sexual patron–client relationships, appear to be increasing as a result of the economic crisis.[34]

The pattern of infection showed a movement of the virus from trading centres into the cities, and outward to the countryside. Women in the rural areas were at risk of infection from migrant husbands returning from the mines or the cities where they had other sexual partners. In the case of migrating husbands, fluid domestic and sexual arrangements were not uncommon. War, destabilization, and displacement were also fuelling the spread of HIV, and the dominant epidemiological paradigm in Africa that focused on female 'prostitutes' effectively left out not only the many contexts of transactional sex, but also the gender dynamics underpinning women's risk of infection, who were displaced or caught up in armed conflict and political violence. The forcible abduction and rape of women were the direct consequences of war, but breakdown of community networks and household cohesion were also pushing women into risk situations.[35] Studies also examined women's ability to protect themselves and to negotiate behavioural change. The conclusions of ethnographic research carried out pointed to the discrepancies between certain groups of women's knowledge about AIDS and their ability to negotiate about behaviour change with their partners. It was becoming clearer that high levels of knowledge about HIV did not correlate with the ability or power to protect oneself from infection.

The impact

It was also becoming clearer that AIDS epidemics were rendering people more vulnerable to other viruses and opportunistic infections, and were putting severe strains on the already grossly insufficient health care systems. In Uganda, Kenya, and Tanzania, AIDS patients were overwhelming hospitals and clinics, and already inadequate supplies of basic drugs could not keep up with the demand created by opportunistic infections. HIV infection was held largely responsible for the resurgence of Tuberculosis (TB). But throughout the 1990s, it was becoming clearer that AIDS was having an impact in countries reaching far beyond family tragedy and strains on the health care sector. Another branch of research that developed focused on the socio-economic impact of AIDS on African economies.

A number of AIDS Assessment and Planning Studies commissioned by the WB examined the impact of AIDS on various sectors of society. By 1990, the United Nations Food and Agricultural Organization (FAO) was predicting AIDS-induced declines in agricultural production. In the agricultural sector, AIDS was having an impact on labour supply and remittance income, leading to significant declines in household production.[36] The International Labour Organization (ILO) looked at labour force impacts, and enterprise and macroeconomic performance, in 2000 estimating a drop in the growth of 25 per cent over a 20-year period in high-prevalence countries, with labour forces in the year 2020 estimated to be between 10 and 22 per cent smaller.[37] Research also focused on the mounting impact of the epidemic on the social sector – increased dependency ratios and the growing number of orphans, shortages of teachers, and health care and other professionals were taxing already beleaguered social services. By the close of the 1990s, echoes of crisis in Africa were heard once again, this time with reference to AIDS-induced famine in many areas of SSA. According to the FAO, 39 per cent of people in the region are malnourished, and predictions are that Africa as a whole would see an increase in food insecurity by 2010.[38] The Chief of the Population Programme Service, Women and Population Division of FAO's Sustainable Development Programme, posed the following questions:

> Can agricultural policies have a significant impact either on the spread and the level of the HIV/AIDS pandemic or on mitigating its impacts? If yes, should national agricultural policies and programmes be used to combat the pandemic actively? If yes, what policy instruments would be effective in the field of agriculture? Such questions have not yet really been explored, and it is understandable that a sectoral ministry might be reluctant to involve itself in an area that it would feel ill-equipped to deal with and that could be defined as coming under the exclusive authority of the Ministry of Health.[39]

Indeed, AIDS has played a role in exacerbating continuing famine in Lesotho, Malawi, Mozambique, Swaziland, Zambia, and Zimbabwe, where as of September 2002, an estimated 14 million were at risk of starvation, according to UN estimates. The spread of AIDS is understood as a 'root cause' for the decline in agricultural production. UNAIDS announced in June 2002:

> Hunger and AIDS are threatening sub-Saharan Africa on two fronts, working in tandem to endanger millions of lives and drive back development ... because of AIDS, farming skills have been lost, agricultural extension services have declined, rural livelihoods have disintegrated, productive capacity to work the land has dropped, and household earnings are shrinking while the cost of caring for the ill skyrockets. [40]

The current crisis is understood principally in terms of a crisis in the supply of domestic farm labour and in the diversion of labour away from subsistence production to caring for the sick. Combining with erratic rainfall, AIDS-related mortality has decimated agricultural labour forces and has left huge numbers of grandparents and orphans to fend for themselves. Furthermore, hunger is pushing people into risky survival strategies, including the selling of sex, further fuelling the epidemic. Other consequences include an increase in migration as impoverished rural dwellers seek opportunities in the cities and towns, maintaining the vicious circle of viral spread.

But the main focus of concern is on declines in gross national product (GNP), exports, and production targets. Less concern is expressed for the intensification of women's unwaged labour and the deepening of poverty in AIDS-affected households. Women's subsistence production remains the taken-for-granted and 'cost-effective' underpinning of the monetized economy. Not to minimize the relationship between famine and AIDS, but it is worth pointing out that AIDS has articulated with underlying structural inequalities that were well entrenched long before the AIDS pandemic to render rural livelihoods tenuous, a history that pre-dates AIDS by decades. Since the 1960s, per capita food production has fallen by about 20 per cent, the only region in the world to experience such a fall.[41] AIDS-induced famine is far more than the inevitable confluence of disease and drought on the African continent.

Many studies illustrate how women's pre-colonial usufruct rights which guaranteed women's independent access to land and the products of their labour were undermined, first by colonial land policies and then by development projects that allocated land ownership to men.[42] It is fair to say that the direct and indirect policies of colonial governments had an overall detrimental effect on women's capacity to maintain their position of relative autonomy within the political economy of the societies in question. As agriculture was commercialized under colonialism, men translated their control over land use into control over the proceeds of cash cropping. In many countries, vast per centages of the total land under cultivation were alienated to non-Africans – to corporate-owned plantations and smaller settler commercial farms. The overall land and time devoted to subsistence production dropped, and were less nutritious, but more efficiently produced staples were introduced as a response to women's increased time burdens. Agricultural production in many African contexts has been tenuous for a long time.

The research on rural women in post-colonial Africa points to the fact that their labour has only intensified, and it has become increasingly difficult for them to feed their families. The circumstances that have led to the 'AIDS and famine crisis' are complex. But certainly what must be considered is the historical relationship between the imposition of export monoculture and the decline in subsistence production and small-scale farming; the effects of agricultural pricing policies and the severe cost/price squeeze felt by some local farmers; the impacts of the instability of international commodity markets on African farmers who are price takers; and the relationship between the dependence of African governments on crop exports for foreign exchange and debt repayment.[43] Scholars working from a feminist perspective have documented the absence of support services and inputs directed at women farmers, and their increasingly tenuous position with regard to access to arable land. Others have analyzed the intensification of women's labour that accompanied austerity measures and its contribution to their decreased ability to feed their families. Erratic rainfall, drought, and soil depletion have also contributed. AIDS intersects with, exacerbates, these trends. A focus on the virus in the absence of a consideration of broader structural inequalities and reigning policy frameworks obscures other contributors to 'the crisis'.

Less research has been carried out on the tangible effects of the epidemic on households, on people's lives. In 1992, *AIDS in Africa: Its Present and Future Impact* was published, representing one of the first comprehensive examinations of the socio-economic impact of the epidemic on an African community. Initially commissioned as an Overseas Development Agency (ODA) study, Barnett and Blaikie analyzed the impact of AIDS on farming systems in the Rakai District of Uganda, and the responses of households and kinship networks.[44] The very small body of descriptive research that has followed, devoted to conditions in rural areas, points to the reality that many of the women who have borne the hidden burden of the epidemic – caring for the sick, making up for shortfalls in labour when family members died – were beyond coping. Researchers at the Uganda Virus Research Institute (UVRI) came to similar conclusions, challenging the assumption of the traditional extended family system as the safety net for individuals, based on their study of rural southwest Uganda.[45] A recent case study of Zimbabwe concluded that older women constitute 60 per cent of those caring for orphans and people with AIDS, and that they are unrewarded, unsupported, lacking the very basics in terms of food, clothing, medical care, and economic support.[46] Reporting on a pilot project in Tanzania, a team of researchers explored the daily lives of 21 caregivers – fifteen women and six men – to 51 AIDS patients. They state that men were involved only when no sister, wife, mother, or daughter was available. All were coping with minimal assistance from neighbours and self-supporting women's and religious associations in the form of food, soap, fetching water and firewood, cleaning, and cooking. At the terminal stage, caring for patients became a full-time job, with no time left for essential tasks such as cultivation.

AIDS and security

> AIDS can no longer be understood or responded to as primarily a public health crisis. It is becoming a threat to security.[47]

The United Nations held a special session at the UN Security Council in January 2000 on AIDS and international security and in May 2000, the Clinton Administration formally designated the spread of AIDS around the world as a threat to its national security. According to Nicholas Eberstadt, a researcher with the American Enterprise Institute,

> so far in Sub-Saharan Africa we've had a catastrophe of world historical proportion. It's been treated as a tragedy, but mainly a humanitarian tragedy. And that's because Sub-Saharan Africa has been essentially marginal to the international economy and the international balance of power ... it becomes an issue as it spreads to countries of strategic proportions to the U.S.[48]

The security threat is understood in different ways. According to the International Crisis Group, AIDS is an international security issue 'both by its potential to contribute to international security challenges, and by its ability to undermine international capacity to resolve conflicts'.[49] The virus, spreading unchecked, threatens to destabilize national armies, and to depress the economies of whole continents, and to kill off the next generation of leaders and skilled workers. Deaths, particularly among the elite, are seen as rendering African countries more difficult to govern. Of particular concern are the high levels of HIV infection amongst military forces, levels reportedly five times that of civilian populations in some armies. Not only does

AIDS threaten to weaken national defence, it also has the potential for limiting peacekeeping operations. The millions of orphans on the continent also pose a security risk as they can be potentially incorporated as child soldiers into rebel groups. And there is mounting evidence that soldiers who are infected engage in risky and even criminal behaviour, using sexual violence as part of their effort to maintain control over civilians and territory, further spreading the virus.

In this post-9/11 world, 'Africa' is now seen as a haven for potential terrorist cells, given its porous borders, weak governance, poor intelligence, and now, rampant HIV infection. The terrorist attacks on the US Embassies in Nairobi and Dar es Salaam in August 1988 and the more recent suicide bombing of Israeli tourists at a resort in Mombassa in November 2002 have placed Africa on the map as a potential haven for extremists. George Bush has expressed a commitment to African economic development as part of US national interests: 'A growing African economy and regional stability enhance the economic prosperity and national security of the United States and the spread of democratic values.' As Leonce Ndikumana asserts, 'The Bush administration seems to understand that with the increased threat of global terrorism, the US cannot afford to ignore an entire continent.'[50]

As with 'AIDS and famine', the dominant discourse on 'AIDS and security' sidelines the material conditions that have perpetuated and continue to perpetuate war and violent conflict, which have been a persistent part of the sub-continent's colonial and post-colonial history. Instability owes much to the legacy of colonialism; the artificiality of arbitrarily imposed national boundaries, colonial policies of divide-and-rule; in the post-colonial present, economic stagnation underlies ethnic cleavages. The unquestioned legitimacy attributed to African uniformed forces as the protectors of national sovereignty and keepers of the peace is a necessary myth to uphold, to justify on the one hand, continued trade in armaments from Europe and North America and, on the other, the strategic military protection of multinational oil and mineral interests on the sub-continent. Some scholars have illustrated how the imposition of structural adjustment and the privatization of the state have reinforced, in many cases, a culture of institutional neglect and the systematic plunder of national resources by elites. Corrupt and autocratic leadership is upheld by military power.[51] It is not clear, in many contexts, whose security armies are protecting.

Others offer more nuanced versions of the crisis of AIDS and security – Oxfam for example, linking 'security' not to global instability and a threat to US national interest, but to a local crisis in food security with severe long-term consequences. Oxfam points directly to unfair international trade regimes, failing agricultural policies, collapsing public services, and crippling debt as contributing to the present crisis and calls for the implementation of sound policies to improve the food security of the most vulnerable people. Among its policy recommendations, it includes the following:

> At the international level, the EU, US, and other rich countries must end double standards in trade policy, radically reducing their massive subsidies to agricultural exports. At the same time they should support the right of developing countries to protect and support their agricultural sectors on the basis of food security and rural development. The US government must stop exerting bilateral pressure on developing countries to introduce unnecessarily high standards of patent protection on medicines. Such pressure restricts and delays the production of cheaper generic medicines, with potentially devastating consequences for millions of poor people.[52]

The dominant framework within which AIDS is understood as a security issue is not Oxfam's, however. How the new understanding of AIDS as a security threat will be reflected in policy still remains to be seen.

AIDS and human rights

The AIDS crisis in Africa is also increasingly viewed through the prism of human rights. According to Sofia Gruskin and Daniel Tarantola, both affiliated with the Francois-Xavier Bagnoud Center for Health and Human Rights, the HIV/AIDS pandemic was a catalyst for beginning to define some of the structural connections between health and human rights:

> the development of a 'health and human rights' language in the last few years has allowed for the connections between health and human rights to be explicitly named, and therefore, for conceptual, analytical, policy and programmatic work to begin to bridge these disparate disciplines and to move forward. In the last few years,

human rights have increasingly been at the centre of analysis and action in regard to health and development issues. The level of institutional and stated political commitment to health and human rights has, in fact, never been higher. This is true within the work of the United Nations system but even more importantly, can also be seen in the work of governments and non-governmental organizations (NGOs) at both the national and international level.[53]

This deeper understanding of AIDS was reflected in the discourse on 'AIDS and human rights', apparent, for example, in the UNAIDS report on the Global HIV/AIDS epidemic 2002:

> HIV/AIDS has burrowed deeper into the social and economic fault lines of communities and societies, and it is widening those fissures further. Around the world, the most affected by HIV/AIDS are people and communities who have unequal access to fundamental social and economic rights. The denial of basic rights limits people's options to defend their autonomy, develop viable livelihoods, and protect themselves, leaving them more vulnerable to both HIV infection and the impact of the epidemic on their lives.[54]

The 'right to health' had been encoded in international law through various mechanisms, beginning with the Universal Declaration of Human Rights in 1948 and more than twenty multilateral treaties since then, which have created legally binding obligations on the part of the signatories. In all, there are 47 conventions dealing with human rights, including those associated with regional organizations and specialized agencies. Conventions are pledges by national authorities to treat nationals in a certain way: in international law, states are the subjects and citizens are the objects. They remain substantially un-enforced. Today, contemporary structures and institutions of governance transcend the nation-state, and an increasingly wide variety of transnational and global actors share the task, including the WTO, the IMF, and the WB, which are not subject to binding human rights legislation, despite the fact that their policies have been linked to the undermining of the exercise of basic human rights. Nor are corporations held accountable for their rights violations. Multilateral agreements on trade, services, and intellectual property on the other hand are binding and are backed up by strong enforcement mechanisms.

Institutions like the WB view the capacity of individual nation-states to protect the human rights of its citizens as dependent on economic growth, trade liberalization, and attracting foreign investment. Given that the protection of human rights is viewed overwhelmingly as the responsibility of the nation-state, African countries are viewed as not able to fulfil their human rights obligations because of low levels of development.

Although the UNAIDS report on AIDS and Human Rights reiterates that in the context of HIV/AIDS, governments have the obligation to respect, protect, and fulfil human rights through the framework of international human rights instruments, the 'right to the highest attainable standard of physical and mental health' is collapsed to ensuring that HIV-prevention tools are available, as well as voluntary testing and counselling, drugs, and necessary health infrastructure and personnel. The onus is on states alone to pursue policies that promote the availability of HIV/AIDS-related medications and 'to protect people who are most vulnerable and disempowered'. As Heywood states: 'It is this unresolved and deepening tension that is arguably now at the crux of global health or ill-health – because what is attainable on the basis of national resources is not the same as what is attainable on the basis of international resources.'[55]

Despite the more inclusive and nuanced understanding of 'African AIDS', the overwhelming focus remains on biology and behaviour. In most of the research on AIDS in Africa, the 'virus' takes on a particular agency that masks other contributors to the 'crisis' – such as debt, privatization and other structural adjustments, falling non-oil commodity prices, and western agricultural subsidies. Also erased is historical context. The virus is seen as undermining the 'impressive strides in human development' that have occurred since the 1960s.

> Countries that fail to bring the epidemic under control risk becoming locked in a vicious circle as worsening socioeconomic conditions render people, enterprises and communities even more vulnerable to the epidemic. The impact of AIDS on societies and economies, however, can be dealt with. Whether through community action or national programmes, institutions can be re-tooled and capacity can be built to defend societies' from the worst ravages of AIDS.[56]

How has the understanding of 'African AIDS' shaped the policy response? It is to this question that I now turn.

Notes

1. Byron Good, *Medicine, Rationality, Experience: An Anthropological Perspective* (Cambridge: Cambridge University Press, 1994) 8.
2. Paul Starr, *The Social Transformation of American Medicine* (New York: Basic Books, 1982) 4.
3. Ibid., 181.
4. Lesley Doyal, *The Political Economy of Health* (Great Britain: Pluto Press, 1979) 33.
5. T. Barnett and A. Whiteside, *AIDS in the Twenty-First Century: Disease and Globalization* (Basingstoke: Palgrave Macmillan, 2002) 27.
6. J. Robinson, *Prescription Games* (Toronto: McClelland and Stewart, 2001) 14.
7. Gerald M. Oppenheimer, 'Causes, Cases and Cohorts: The Role of Epidemiology in the Historical Construction of AIDS', *AIDS: The Making of a Chronic Disease*, eds Elizabeth Fee and Daniel Fox (Berkeley: University of California Press, 1992) 49.
8. Nancy Krieger, 'Epidemiology and the Web of Causation: Has Anyone Seen the Spider?' *Social Science and Medicine* 39 (1994): 887.
9. Steven Epstein, *Impure Science: AIDS, Activism and the Politics of Knowledge* (Berkeley: University of California Press, 1996) 50.
10. Oppenheimer, 270–82.
11. Farmer, *Infections* 62.
12. Epstein, 25.
13. Ibid., 32.
14. Ibid.,65.
15. Ibid., 55.
16. Ibid., 21.
17. Simon Watney, *Practices of Freedom: Selected Writings on HIV/AIDS* (London: Meuthen, 1994) 11.
18. Jeff O'Malley, 'AIDS Service Organizations in Transition', *AIDS in the World*, eds. Mann *et al.* (Cambridge: Harvard University Press, 1992) 777.
19. See, for example, UNAIDS, *A Human Rights Approach to AIDS Prevention at Work: The Southern African Development Community's Code on HIV/AIDS and Employment* (Geneva: UNAIDS, 2000).
20. Nancy Scheper-Hughes, 'AIDS and the Social Body', *Social Science and Medicine* 39 (1994): 992.
21. Paul Farmer, *Pathologies of Power: Health, Human Rights, and the New War on the Poor* (Berkeley: University of California Press, 2003) 162.
22. A. Ona Pela and Jerome J. Platt, 'AIDS in Africa: Emerging Trends', *Social Science and Medicine* 28.1 (1989): 1–8.
23. Brooke Grundfest Schoepf, 'Political Economy, Sex and Cultural Logics: A View from Zaire', unpublished paper, subsequently published as B. G. Schoepf, 'Political Economy, Sex and Cultural Logics: A View from Zaire', *African Urban Quarterly* 6.1–2 (1991): 94–106.
24. See, for example, D. Serwadda, 'Slim Disease: A New Disease in Uganda and its Association with HTLV-III Infection', *The Lancet* 19 (1985): 849–52; Peter Piot *et al.*, 'Heterosexual Transmission of HIV', *AIDS* 1 (1987): 199–206;

J. Killewo *et al.*, eds, 'Behavioural and Epidemiological Aspects of AIDS Research in Tanzania', workshop proceedings (Dar es Salaam, Tanzania: 6–8 Dec. 1989).

25. See, for example, Judith E. Brown, Okako B. Ayowa, and Richard C. Brown, 'Dry and Tight: Sexual Practices and Potential AIDS Risk in Zaire', *Social Science and Medicine* 37.8 (1993): 989–94.

26. Douglas Feldman, 'Editorial', *Social Science and Medicine* 33.7 (1991): 784.

27. Angela Molnos, ed., *Cultural Source Materials for Population Planning in East Africa*, Vol. 2 (Nairobi: East African Publishing House, 1972) 19.

28. Brooke G. Schoepf, 'Ethical, Methodological and Political Issues of AIDS Research in Central Africa', *Social Science and Medicine* 33.7 (1991): 752.

29. Eileen Stillwaggon, 'HIV/AIDS in Africa: Fertile Terrain', *Journal of Development Studies* 38.6 (2002): 17.

30. Helen Epstein, 'AIDS: The Lesson of Uganda', *New York Review of Books* (15 July 2001): 20.

31. D. Frommel, 'Editorial', *Le Monde Diplomatique English Supplement to the Guardian* (Jan. 2001): 11.

32. Tony Barnett and Piers Blaikie, *AIDS in Africa: Its Present and Future Impact* (London: Belhaven Press, 1992).

33. Mary Bassett and Marvellous Mhloyi, 'Women and AIDS in Zimbabwe: The Making of an Epidemic', *International Journal of Health Services* 21.1 (1991): 143–46.

34. Brooke G. Schoepf, 'Action Research on Women in Kinshasa: Community-based Risk Reduction Support', unpublished report (1992): 4.

35. See, for example, Gill Seidel, 'Women at Risk: Gender and AIDS in Africa', *Disasters* 17.2 (1993): 133–42.

36. UNAIDS/FAO, 'HIV/AIDS Epidemic is Shifting from Cities to Rural Areas: New Focus on Agricultural Policy Needed', Press release (Rome-Geneva: UNAIDS, 22 June 2000).

37. International Labour Organization, 'AIDS a Major Threat to the World of Work' (ILO, 8 June 2000) (http://www.ilo.org/public/english/protetion/trav/aids/index.htm).

38. FAO, 'Food Supply Situation and Crop Prospects in Sub-Saharan Africa No. 3' (FAO, Dec. 2002) (ftp://ftp.fao.org/docrep/fao/005/y2916e00.pdf).

39. J. du Guernny, 'AIDS and Agriculture in Africa: Can Agricultural Policy Make a Difference?' *Food, Nutrition and Agriculture* 25 (1999): 16 (ftp://ftp.fao.org/docrep/fao/X4390t/X4390t03.pdf).

40. UNAIDS News Dispatch, 'Africa Faces Dual Tragedy as Famine and AIDS Strike in Tandem' (Rome: UNAIDS, 12 June 2002).

41. Jules Pretty, 'Can Sustainable Agriculture Feed Africa? New Evidence on Progress, Processes, and Impact', *Environment, Development and Sustainability* 1.3/4 (1999): 253–74.

42. See, for example, Carolyn Clark, 'Land and Food, Women and Power in Nineteenth Century Kikuyu', *Africa* 50.4 (1980): 359–69; Jane Guyer, 'Female Farming and the Evolution of Food Production Patterns Amongst the Beti of South Central Cameroon', *Africa* 50.4 (1980): 341–55; Elias Mandala, 'Peasant Cotton Agriculture, Gender and Inter-generational

Relationships: The Lower Tchiri Valley of Malawi, 1906–1940', *African Studies Review* 25.2/3 (1982): 27–43; Maud Muntemba, 'Women and Agricultural Change in the Railway Region of Zambia: Dispossession and Counterstrategies, 1930–1970', *Women and Work in Africa*, ed. Edna Bay (Boulder: Westview Press, 1982): 83–106; Sherilynn Young, 'Fertility and Famine: Women's Agricultural History in Southern Mozambique', *The Roots of Rural Poverty in Central and Southern Africa*, eds Robin Palmer and Neil Parsons (Berkeley: University of California Press, 1977): 66–81.

43. See, for example, Peter Lawrence, ed., *World Recession and the Food Crisis in Africa* (London: James Currey, 1986), which examines the complex contemporary history of Sub-Saharan Africa's agricultural crisis.

44. Barnett and Blaikie.

45. J. Seeley *et al.*, 'Family Support for AIDS Patients in a Rural Population in Southwest Uganda: How Much a Myth?', unpublished paper, Medical Research Council (MRC) (UK) Programme on AIDS in Uganda (Entebbe: MRC/UVRI, 1992).

46. WHO, 'Impact of AIDS on Older People in Africa' (Geneva: WHO, Dec. 2002) (http://www.who.int/hpr/ageing/zimaidsreport.pdf).

47. International Crisis Group, *HIV/AIDS as a Security Issue* (Washington/ Brussels: ICG, 19 June 2001) (http://www.intl-crisis-group.org/projects/ issues/hiv_aids/reports/A400321_190602001.pdf).

48. Nicholas Eberstadt qtd in PBS Online News Hour, 'AIDS Threatens Global Security' (PBS, 1 Oct. 2002) <http://www.pbs.org/newshour/bb/inter- national/july_dec02/aids_10_01.html>.

49. International Crisis Group.

50. Léonce Ndikumana, 'Beyond Good Intentions: Is U.S. Newly found interest in Africa real?' *Econ-Atrocity Bulletin* (22 Jan. 2003) (http://www.fguide.org/ Bulletin/africa.htm).

51. See, for example, Jean-Francois Bayart, Stephen Ellis, and Beatrice Hibou, *The Criminalization of the State in Africa* (Oxford: James Currey, 1999); Bonny Ibhawoh, 'Structural Adjustment, Authoritarianism, and Human Rights in Africa', *Comparative Studies of South Asia, Africa and the Middle East* XIX.1 (1999): 158–67.

52. Oxfam International, *HIV/AIDS and Food Insecurity in Southern Africa* (Oxfam, 1 Dec. 2002) 5 (http://www.oxfam.org/eng/pdfs/pp021127_ aids_Safrica.pdf).

53. Sofia Gruskin and Daniel Tarantola, *Health and Human Rights*, Francois- Xavier Bagnoud Center Working Paper No. 10 (Boston: FXB Center, 2000): 1 (http://www.hsph.harvard.edu/fxbcenter/FXBC_WP10–Gruskin_and_ Tarantola.pdf).

54. UNAIDS, 'Focus: AIDS and Human Rights', *Report on the Global HIV/AIDS Epidemic 2002*: 62 <http://www.unaids.org/barcelona/preskit/barcelona%20 report/focus_ humanrights.pdf>.

55. Mark Heywood, 'Drug Access, Patents and Global Health: "Chaffed and Waxed Sufficient"', *Third World Quarterly* 23.2 (2002): 219.

56. UNAIDS, 'Focus' 44.

2
Africa in the Global Institutional Response

This chapter focuses on the ways in which SSA has been cast in the global institutional response to the AIDS pandemic, with particular attention to the ideological meanings and policy directions attached to neoliberal restructuring, and the ways in which they have conditioned the response on the ground. In the previous chapter, I argued that a multidimensional understanding of African AIDS has emerged over the past two decades – one that goes beyond a narrow focus on the behavioural and biological, and considers broader structural factors such as poverty, migration, instability, and unequal gender relations in shaping the pattern of HIV spread, and illuminates the broad impacts of AIDS on various sectors beyond health. How has that understanding conditioned the policy response in SSA?

The complex contradictions embodied in the practices of development assistance are perhaps nowhere more difficult to untangle than in Africa. As the continent that remains the most marginalized in the global economy according to all indicators, be they macroeconomic or human development, it is also the place most subject to the dictates of donors – in today's language, 'development partners' – in part owing to the AIDS pandemic. The institutional response to AIDS has been executed by a diverse range of actors and agencies, from the very local to the global. These agencies operate within the constraints imposed by the imperatives of global neoliberal restructuring, in some cases entrenching and in other cases contesting certain policies and practices. African leaders are not without agency; they can determine whether or not to confront HIV epidemics within their borders. And people on the ground can twist and bend the constraints imposed upon them. But the room for manoeuvre is circumscribed by a wide range of factors: by conditionalities set by donor agencies; by limited financial resources in turn related to broader socio-economic factors including debt; and by state capacity to influence the policy agenda and to monitor AIDS-related interventions through their national AIDS commissions or secretariats. The role of states is to coordinate and to oversee the activities of a broad range of institutions, both local and foreign, while NGOs, consultants, 'communities', and the private sector implement policies and projects, in some cases acting as the foreign policy instruments of donor states. NGOs and the private sector have moved in where the state has left off in the provision of health care and other social welfare services.

Various clusters of power in the 'AIDS and development' world began to evolve around the mid-1980s. At the centre was the UN, with WHO taking the lead role but other UN agencies, in particular, UNICEF, United Nations Development Programme (UNDP), and the WB, participating in the WHO/GPA and also developing their own AIDS programmes. The United States through United States Agency for International Development (USAID) was the largest single bilateral donor in Africa, but other bilateral donors participated through the support of the GPA or through their own programmes. Thousands of CSOs, local and foreign, have projects in SSA and since the 1990s, the private sector has taken on an increasingly significant role. The WHO/GPA led the global institutional response from 1986 onwards, taking the professional and technical lead in establishing AIDS programmes in its member countries, and a general consensus developed among the major powers on how the pandemic would be managed. Most donor governments gave unanimous support to WHO's strategy for encouraging countries to set up National AIDS Programmes. The GPA became an important mechanism of coordination for countries receiving development assistance, and financial support for AIDS Control Programmes depended on each recipient country developing a plan, programme, and staff committed to combating the spread of AIDS.

The boundaries are blurred among the various participants in the continually evolving AIDS industry. Multilateral and bilateral funding is often channelled through NGOs, and 'partnerships' between government ministries, NGOs, and the private sector are increasingly common. In what follows, I make an attempt to illuminate the main features and activities of the various actors and their relationship to one another – states, multilateral institutions, bilateral donors, CSOs, and the private sector – drawing out what have been the most significant elements of the policy response over the last decade, and their political and institutional contexts. The next chapter focuses specifically on the politics of vaccine research and pharmaceutical provision, while this chapter focuses on the main policy responses with regard to prevention, care, and mitigating impacts. I begin, though, with a brief background on the broader political/economic context.

The context: Africa's lost decades

The beginning of Africa's crisis is generally dated to the continent's entanglement in unsustainable levels of debt precipitated by the global economic recession and the downward spiral of world commodity prices during the late 1970s and early 1980s. Many fragile, newly independent states became increasingly obliged to 'adjust' their economies to a severely unstable and complex environment of oil shocks and deteriorating terms of trade. The economic problems of African countries in these years were hardly brand new; colonial policy had forged a regime of primary resource extraction for export to the detriment of local development and food production for local consumption. The global economic recession had a disproportionate effect on the African continent, given its dependence on primary products for export. Africa's first 'lost decade' was the 1980s. Peter Lawrence wrote in 1985:

> By any estimation, SSA is in a state of profound economic, social and political crisis. Growth rates have declined sharply since 1973 in all sectors and have been outstripped or matched by rising population growth rates. Food production per capita has fallen over the last decade by up to 15 per cent in some countries and 6 per cent over the whole of the region. Cereal imports have risen by 117 per cent and food imports by 172 per cent.[1]

The 1980s ushered in the stabilization and adjustment programmes of the IMF and the WB. The IMF was responsible for short-term stabilization programmes, and the WB oriented towards increasing supply-side efficiency and stimulating productive investment. Stabilization induced adjustment mainly through demand effects, though policies of fiscal and monetary restraint such as deflation and currency devaluation.

Cutting public expenditure, loosening control over foreign imports and exchange, increasing incentives for private-sector producers (particularly exports) through changes in prices, tariffs, taxes, subsidies, and interest rates, and reducing resources allocated to the public sector were the policies characteristic of stabilization. Stabilization was meant to reduce real incomes and hence domestic demand for imports and exports, thereby reducing countries' import bills, and expanding their exports. The establishment of this regime was conditional on the granting of loans. Structural adjustment emphasized the supply side, and was meant to tackle balance of payment problems by expanding and diversifying the production of exports, enabling a country to cope with the vagaries of the unstable global environment by increasing productivity and efficiency, and by shifting to the production of goods with better growth prospects. Resources were to be channelled into regions with high growth potential and were to be focused on large, successful farmers. The original blueprint for conditionality, the World Bank Report 'Accelerated Development in Sub-Saharan Africa' written in 1981, outlined the basic policy prescription: a shift in internal trade towards exporters, the trimming of the state and the encouragement of privatization, cuts in urban real wages, and the establishment of user fees for state-provided services.

The implicit assumption of macroeconomic policy is that the processes of reproduction and the maintenance of human life which is carried out largely by unpaid women will continue regardless of the way resources are allocated. Women's unpaid labour was implicitly regarded as infinitely elastic, able to stretch so as to make up any shortfall in other resources available for reproduction. But processes of reproduction, the care of humans, is different from that of the production of any other kind of resource; as Diane Elson eloquently put it, 'if the demand for labour falls, if unemployment rises, if wages decline, mothers do not "scrap" their children or leave them to rot unattended in the fields'.[2] What was regarded as increased 'efficiency' by economists was the shifting of costs away from the formal economy and the state to the subsistence sector and to women. The reduction in the time spent by patients in hospital – measured as an increase in 'efficiency' – was an invisible cost borne largely by women. In 1988, UNICEF documented the widespread deterioration in the health of children and pregnant and lactating mothers in both rural and urban areas in 'stabilizing' regions, pointing to the IMF/WB conditionality as being responsible for the deaths of half-a-million children.[3]

The wider causes and consequences of Africa's continued state of 'crisis' and its apparent intractability have been debated and analyzed in detail. The WB and the IMF have consistently attributed Africa's crisis to domestic policy issues; overvalued exchange rates, inappropriate agricultural policies, excessive state intervention, and costly import substitution. By the end of the 1980s, the focus was also on corrupt, and autocratic governments and political conflict; Africa could pull itself out of poverty through 'good governance', the new carrot of aid and loan conditionality. By the end of the 1980s, the WB had moved beyond its original mandate of economic reform to redefining the role and function of the African state and promoting a distinct role for state–market relations. The state's role, according to the Bank, is to contribute to the creation of a policy environment favourable to open economies and free markets, and to intervene to correct market failures. Its role in redistribution, in the provision of basic services, is conditional upon its capacity to carry out its primary economic function – to stimulate growth.[4] It is not clear which states are accountable for – their constituencies or global creditors. While prescribing open markets for African states, the international trade machinery has continued to operate against African exports; while insisting that African countries should withdraw their farm subsidies, OECD countries have regularly increased theirs. The concerns of African leaders were ignored at the WTO's Doha meeting in November 2001 and have been so since.[5] Rich countries of the north continue to spend vast amounts subsidizing their farmers – Carol Thompson puts the figure at $1 billion a day – an annual subsidy three times as large as the entire amount spent on development assistance.[6]

Instead of a market-based economic and social recovery, Africa has instead fallen further into debt and disorder. Certainly not all of Africa's woes can be attributed to neoliberalism – Africa's underdevelopment is a function of the consequences of both colonialism and present-day neocolonialism, and corrupt politics and failed leadership; the two not unrelated. Many scholars[7] have analyzed the connections between privatization and adjustment policies, the rise of authoritarianism, and, in some polities, the 'criminalization of the behaviour of power holders'.[8]

With South Africa providing the only really important exception, the process of democracy has been captured under the guise of competitive elections, by the authoritarian groups already in control of state power (notably Cote d'Ivoire, Togo, Cameroon, Gabon and Kenya), or it has given rise to new regimes whose weakness offers little promise of future stability (Mali and Benin) or produced others which cannot be considered genuinely democratic (Central African Republic, Congo until 1997, Equatorial Guinea, Zambia, Chad) or else democracy has been snuffed out by intervention of armed forces (Nigeria, Niger, Burundi). Efforts to combine the requirements of a market economy with the demands of popular sovereignty have ended in failure.[9]

Indeed, it is the case that certain polities can be accurately described as mafias – Somalia, Liberia, Sierra Leone, Democratic Republic of the Congo (DRC) – whose leaders are military entrepreneurs amassing vast wealth in foreign bank accounts; others are more benign, benefiting from control over the management of imports, overwhelmingly consumer rather than capital goods, as one of the few available sites of accumulation of wealth and power.[10] Vast amounts of plundered wealth have been deposited in foreign bank accounts, while debt has increased. But none of this has happened without western complicity, and some commentators have pointed to the relationship between privatization and the plunder of state resources, as well as the authoritarian nature of the imposition of structural adjustment programmes. Ann Pettifor comments on the international complicity that made possible the plunder of Zaire by its former ruler Mobutu – his personal fortune estimated at between two and twelve billion when he died in 1998. As early as 1974, there were clear warnings that loans were being stolen, but Zaire's creditors continued lending and kept him in power with western arms. The cost of unwise and corrupt borrowing has not been borne by elites or western creditors, but has resulted in further immiseration and disempowerment of the poorest.

With the new millennium came a new global compact adopted by 189 countries to halve extreme poverty, halt the spread of HIV/AIDS, and enrol all children in primary school by 2015 – the Millennium Development Goals. Based on the indicators from the UN Development Report 2003, there seems little hope for African countries reaching the goals despite a few 'success stories' – Uganda, Senegal, and Ghana. Of 54 countries that grew poorer over the last decade, 20 were in SSA, and others showing marginal improvement have deep pockets of entrenched poverty. Thirty of thirty-four countries classified as low human development are in SSA.[11] States the report: 'Almost across the board, the story is one of stagnation. Economies have not grown, half of Africans live in extreme poverty and one-third in hunger, and about one-sixth of children die before the age of five – the same as a decade ago.'[12] The present decade appears to be turning into yet another lost decade for Africa, the place on the globe where extraordinary levels of human suffering and deprivation are seemingly acceptable.

The WHO and international health

The WHO spearheaded the policy response to AIDS in the Third World. Reflected in the WHO/GPA was the basic approach of WHO to health problems in the Third World. WHO was founded as one of the UN's specialized agencies in 1946, its mandate to 'improve the health of the world's inhabitants'. Jeffrey Harrod describes this period as one in which a new hegemony was being established based on the globalization of professional discourse, through the first international conferences on issues such as agriculture, population, human rights, and environment. The emerging global professional discourse was to be codified in UN agencies in a manner which indicated their role in a hegemonic system: the major programmes not only reflected but also promoted the ideas and perceptions necessary to sustain the basic community of the liberal status quo.[13] This was also the time, according to Escobar, that mass poverty in Asia, Africa, and Latin America was 'discovered', providing the anchor for state interventionism within a general model of economic liberalism. Within the general liberal model, economic growth was viewed as the necessary route to human progress, but unprecedented social action was needed to lift up the 'diseased, underfed, uneducated and physiologically weak masses'.[14] The UN organizations reflected the global bureaucratization of social action and the beginnings of the production of comprehensive, integrated, and multisectoral strategies based on rational planning, which have become standard fare. The WHO has worked largely as an advisor to its member states and in fact has never had the budget to do much more. Its influence, however, has been deeply felt. Its initial approach to disease in the Third World was strongly influenced by wartime advances in chemical disease controls, interventions that had been developed to reduce high levels of sickness among troops in Latin America and the Pacific Region. Its approach was heavily biomedical. In an in-depth study of WHO conducted by Harold Jacobson in 1967, all but one of the 33 'core group' of policy formulators within WHO were medical doctors.[15] The influence of national associations of doctors, such as the American Medical Association, ensured that within WHO-sponsored programmes, all medical assistance be given by, or in the presence of, a fully qualified doctor.

This policy was finally broken in the mid-1970s by which time thirteen newly independent states, mainly on the African continent, had become members of WHO. It was increasingly recognized that WHO's programs reflected western public health practices and did not adequately address the needs of developing countries. The 1960s and 1970s saw the development of the principles of Primary Health Care (PHC) and Country Health Programming. PHC was canonized at Alma-Ata – a major WHO/UNICEF conference in 1978 in Kazakhstan, at which the WHO and its member states defined a new constitutional objective, 'the attainment by all citizens of the world by the year 2000 of a level of health which will permit them to lead a socially and economically productive life', and the means of achieving this PHC.[16] The WHO's 'Health for All' campaign was one among four of the UN's declarations of 'new order' formulated in the 1970s, the others being the New International Economic Order of the UN General Assembly, United Nations Conference on Trade and Development (UNCTAD), the New World Information and Communication Order of UNESCO, and an updated World Employment Programme of ILO. The PHC approach embodied the ideas that health depended on improving socio-economic conditions and alleviating poverty, and that the process should be community-based and should support health priorities at a local level. The emphasis of health planning shifted from the construction of hospitals to PHC centres, which were to be decentralized, foster local participation, and use appropriate technology.

The birth of Alma-Ata, however, was quickly followed by its death barely 2 years later, precipitated by the oil and debt crisis on the African continent. Three major policy shifts undermined the essence of PHC and heralded the beginning of Africa's so-called 'lost decade': the introduction of selective PHC in the early 1980s; the push for cost-recovery and user-financed health services introduced in the late 1980s; and finally, the takeover of Third World health-care policy by the WB in the 1990s, all three were a reflection of the underlying macroeconomic and ideological trends.[17] Selective Primary Health Care (SPHC) was introduced in 1984 at a joint Ford and Rockefeller Foundation meeting on health services, a policy designed to prevent or treat the few diseases responsible for the greatest mortality or morbidity in Third World countries. Underlying SPHC was the argument that given economic recession and shrinking health budgets, health indicators would improve only with a few carefully selected, cost-effective, and carefully targeted interventions. The 'twin engines' of SPHC were immunization and oral rehydration therapy for children under five.[18]

Although the practice of PHC was rather short-lived, the discourse did not disappear. On the African continent, it was reflected in cost-recovery schemes such as UNICEF's Bamako Initiative through which consumers of essential drugs at rural health posts were charged reduced prices, just enough to keep the health posts running. Health education and community efforts to enhance basic hygiene and sanitation were also a part of Bamako. Lauded not only as a way to re-establish rural health posts that had been closed due to shrinking health budgets, it was also seen as a means to enhance community participation and self-reliance. Communities insofar as they existed were increasingly fractured by migration in search of subsistence, increased competition for scarce resources, and particularly for women, the intensification of their labour as the means to combat some of the negative effects of the economic crisis. In some high-prevalence regions, particularly the area around Lake Victoria, AIDS was beginning to exact its toll in the mid- to late 1980s.

But ideas of cost recovery, privatization, and self-reliance found their ultimate expression in The WB's 1993 World Bank Development Report (WBDR), *Investing in Health*. This report signalled the WB's emerging interest in global health policy. More significantly, it marked the hijacking of the global health agenda from the WHO. It specifically proposed: the reduction of public expenditures on tertiary facilities, specialist training, and interventions that are not cost-effective; the financing for a select package of public health interventions dealing with infectious disease control and environmental pollution; the financing for a package of essential clinical services for the poor; the promotion of private finance for all clinical services outside the essential package; the encouragement to private suppliers to compete for both the delivery of clinical services and the provision of inputs such as drugs to the public and private sectors, with the protection of domestic suppliers from international competition.[19] Kenna Owoh argues that WBDR not only endorsed the pervasive global strategy of IMF/WB-led structural adjustment programmes, but also contributed to that strategy through the 'systematization of global social welfare'. Not surprisingly, absent from the report is a consideration of how political and economic interests tied to the global adjustment regime contribute to the African health crisis. Owoh states:

> The WB and the IMF are restructuring African economies under SAPs to ensure the ease of entry of TNCs, and to realign African economies in the direction of the new global order. Second, under 'second order' adjustment, social unrest is brought under the global agenda. The areas of state autonomy vis-à-vis global institutions have been progressively limited, starting with the economic and moving to the social, and the role of the state is reduced to overseeing the implementation of the global agenda at the local level.[20]

The WB's health strategy was one instrument for bringing global health policy into line with the neoliberal canon that ascribed health mainly to the private domain, through the introduction of market forces into the health sector and the allocation of public resources according to the criteria of technical efficiency and cost-effectiveness. Investing in low-cost actions that target those living in critical poverty, and promoting diversity and competition by facilitating and overseeing private-sector involvement – a policy consistent with the notion that social welfare is the responsibility of the individual – became one of the roles of the government. The WB's *Investing in Health* also marked a new emphasis in the policy agenda on health care financing reform, a topic Kelly Lee and Hilary Goodman explore in some detail. Mapping health care policy reform through key periods of policy development from Alma-Ata to the Commission on Macroeconomics and Health in 2000, the authors describe the creation of a global 'epistemic community' or policy network with a specific set of technical expertise, 'narrowly based in a small number of institutions, led by the WB and USAID, and in the nationality and disciplinary backgrounds of the key individuals involved'.[21]

> A typical career pattern would be Ph.D. training (usually in economics) and then faculty position in a prominent academic institution; project funding from a donor agency such as USAID or World Bank; move to the donor agency as staff member or technical advisor; and/or recruitment by one of a number of small consultancy firms that have worked closely with donor agencies on health care finance issues.[22]

World Health Organization, the Pan-American Health Organization, and NGOs, the authors claim, have been noticeably absent from this new epistemic community, which in a top-down fashion guides the global health policy agenda; an agenda that focuses less on health care as a universal good which should be accessible to all, and more on health system financing, reflecting the new hegemony of the linguistics of economics in health policy. What also distinguishes this new global health policy elite from previous ones is the mix of public and private interests contained in the institutional structure, and its quite substantial power to determine health funding priorities, given the severe financial and human resource constraints of recipient countries in participating in a meaningful way in the policy dialogue.[23]

Throughout these watersheds, The WHO has more or less consistently put forth a view of health that transcends curative medicine and incorporates an understanding of the wider social constituents of health; within the field of international health many institutions still attempt to practice certain principles of PHC in their programmes and projects, such as decentralized health service delivery and community participation. But the links between the capacity of 'local communities' to guarantee access to the basic constituents of health and the circumstances within which these 'local communities' find themselves are rarely articulated. The power of the UN and particularly WHO has greatly diminished vis-à-vis the WB, which has been instrumental in determining health care agendas over the past two decades, and is also the single largest lender for AIDS prevention in Africa. In a number of editorials published between 1994 and 1997, Fiona Godlee depicts the WHO as 'losing its influence and retreating into its technical and biomedical shell'[24] in part due to an absence of effective leadership, its focus on disease-specific intervention programmes which tend to be top-down vertical interventions as opposed to horizontal strengthening of health care systems, and its focus on special programmes funded by extra-budgetary contributions, which shift the power to donors in the determination of priorities.[25]

The tilt in health governance towards neoliberalism is also reflected in 'a qualitatively new hybrid form of governance'[26] Global Public–Private Partnerships (GPPPs). Through GPPPs, industry has been able to secure its influence in UN decision-making circles, a sentiment echoed by Stephen Lewis, who more forcefully speaks of the UN's 'mindless entente with the private sector'.[27] Certain industries have embarked on a multipronged strategy to gain access to and influence multinational and UN decision-making as a means of establishing the 'global rules for ordered liberalism'.[28] More troubling to many are the partnerships between the UN and transnational corporations (TNCs) under the Global Compact, since its launch by Secretary General Kofi Annan in the summer of 2000. The Compact is made up of nine principles distilled from key environmental human rights and labour agreements that corporate members are asked to voluntarily abide by. Its purpose is to harness the resources of business for sustainable development.[29] Known violators of human rights, and labour and environmental violators have joined, including Shell, Nike, BP Amoco, the British mining corporation Rio Tinto Pic, and Novartis. In the context of shrinking UN budgets, the promise of financial resources offered by TNCs is a strong incentive for partnership. UNAIDS has partnered five pharmaceutical giants to determine ways to render ARVs more affordable in Third World countries, which provides them with good public relations and a platform through which to push their own business agendas regarding global standards and law. (I will have more to say about this in the next chapter.) The Alliance for a Corporate Free UN, a global network of environmental human rights and development groups working to address growing corporate influence in the UN, cautions that the legitimacy derived from the near universal membership of its governing bodies is eroding and that global standards and norms are moving more closely to reflect private interests.[30]

These contextual factors matter deeply. The response to HIV/AIDS in Africa has emerged in this broader context of economic and political crisis: stagnating economic growth, minimal state revenues and critical resource shortages, political instability, and in some cases dysfunctional political systems. Political and economic stagnation has accompanied the increased power of the WB and related communities of experts dominated by economists in shaping the global health agenda, and the increased power and autonomy of global capital vis-à-vis the UN and the nation-state.

The Global Program on AIDS

As early as 1985, the possibility of widespread heterosexual transmission of HIV infection was taken more seriously, with the spread of HIV in Central Africa posing a direct challenge to the 'gay lifestyle' model of HIV transmission. As the epidemics in African countries worsened, attention shifted to AIDS outside North America and Western Europe. The WHO/GPA led the global institutional response from 1986 onward. The GPA became the coordinating and funding mechanism for countries receiving development assistance, making its financial support conditional on each country developing a programme and staff committed to AIDS. The Director General of WHO, Hafdan Mahler, stated in 1987:

> A global problem of this magnitude and broad impact – social, economic, demographic, cultural and political – such a global problem requires a global response ... Just as smallpox eradication only became a reality when the nations banded together under the banner of WHO, so AIDS will require global mobilization around a global strategy.[31]

In April 1986, WHO held the first meeting of donors, bringing together representatives from Europe, the US, Japan, and the WB, and proposed to form a Control Programme on AIDS. Later in the year, the World Health Assembly passed a resolution endorsing a global strategy on AIDS, with the sponsorship from 23 countries. The early activities of the Control Programme on AIDS focused on the exchange of information, preparation and distribution of guidelines and education materials, assessment of diagnostic methodology, advice on the provision of safe blood and blood products, and coordination of biological, epidemiological, and behavioural research, these activities in keeping with WHO's traditional technical assistance. In early 1987, the Control Program on AIDS was given the status of a WHO special programme, and shortly thereafter was renamed the Global Program on AIDS (GPA). The GPA established the criteria to formulate a National AIDS Programme: a National Advisory Committee on AIDS has to be appointed; a programme manager had to be identified; a plan had to be formulated that was consistent with the global strategy approved by member states of the World Health Assembly that included objectives, targets, and an implementation plan; and the programme had to have a budget allocation.[32] By the close of the decade, 159 of 167 member governments of the WHO had received some support from the GPA. The standardized and uncontroversial approach made it possible for the GPA to respond to requests for assistance, and it organized more than 1300 consultant missions between 1988 and 1989.[33]

The first requests for assistance from member countries led to one-year short-term plans. Activities carried out under the umbrella of short-term plans typically included epidemiological surveillance, sensitization of health workers, laboratory strengthening for blood safety and testing, mass media campaigns, and advocacy with national policy-makers. Medium-term plans followed shortly thereafter. The standard goals of most of the original medium-term plans were to prevent the sexual transmission of HIV, to prevent transmission through infected blood and blood products, to prevent mother-to-child transmission, and to reduce the individual and social impact of AIDS. Activities were grouped under four main budgetary headings: programme management, epidemiological surveillance, laboratory support, and health education/Information, Education, Communication (IEC).

The growth of the GPA was, unlike any in the history of the WHO, evolving from a staff of two and a budget of US$1 million in 1986 to a staff of 400 and a budget of nearly US$100 million by early 1990.[34] A number of institutional mechanisms created as part of the GPA brought actors from the biomedical and international development fields together. Two structures were instituted within the GPA for inter-agency coordination; the GPA Management Committee in 1988, consisting of WHO's external partners and performing an external review and monitoring function, and the Inter-agency Advisory Group, organized under the leadership of the GPA and including representatives of all UN agencies with AIDS programmes. As well, the Global Commission on AIDS was established, consisting of 30 people from the medical and public health fields to offer expert guidance on the interpretation of scientific and technical trends, and advice on priorities.

According to Tony Klouda, the GPA initially viewed AIDS as a simple biomedical problem requiring a technical solution: 'National AIDS Programmes were the logical response to that way of thinking, and identical plans – crafted from a position of total ignorance of the unique socio-economic and cultural factors shaping epidemics worldwide – was the tragic outcome.'[35] Indeed, it was the case that the response was weighted heavily towards the biomedical, but the interventions were appropriate. The problem was that they were one-sided. But as well, national AIDS programmes were being implemented by weak ministries of health that were subject to severe resource constraints, both financial and human, which had been further weakened by severe budget cuts under SAPs. Many were struggling with providing the absolute basics and covering their recurrent costs before HIV/ AIDS. The fact that AIDS-specific programmes fared poorly was hardly a surprise given the low level of basic health service provision in general. The fact that preventable and curable conditions such as TB, STDs, malaria, cholera, and measles were widespread reflected the fact that health systems were not meeting basic needs.

Prevention programmes, in the form of IEC also ran into problems from the beginning. They intruded on people's sensibilities, and exposed and made public practices that people, particularly men, did not want to be discussed. Attempts to provide sensitive and culturally specific information through popular theatre and schools seemed to work better than the mass education approach, but the sole focus on education belied the context. For many, AIDS was just one more in a long list of potential life hazards – for people who had lived through war, who had buried family members who had died from one of the many preventable diseases, who were suffering from malnutrition, who were working in high-risk sectors like mining, contracting HIV infection seemed to be the least of their worries.

Like other diseases, HIV spread was fastest amongst marginalized populations, higher rates of infection occurring in places with high levels of poverty and instability. As the socio-economic impact of HIV epidemics began to receive more attention, AIDS was increasingly understood as a problem with many dimensions beyond conventionally defined health. Within the Global Programme, the discourse on AIDS underwent a shift from a predominantly biomedical understanding to one which resonated heavily with the prevailing discourses on community-based development and PHC. Within the WHO/GPA, the multisectoral, multidisciplinary, and global nature of the response that was required was publicly acknowledged.[36] But the main problem was perceived as one of the inability of the WHO to operationalize the multisectoral understanding. There was no shortage of policy pronouncements and rhetorical support for a multisectoral strategy from the GPA. Other UN agencies involved in AIDS policy viewed WHO's approach as too technical and narrowly medical. The External Review Committee of the GPA stated in 1992 that the overall responsibility for planning and coordinating a response would more appropriately lie outside the WHO, and would be better placed under the leadership of the UNDP or the WB.[37] The External Review goes on to say:

> The concept of AIDS as a social, economic and demographic problem as well as a health care issue has been widely recognized at country level but rarely operationalized. The National AIDS Committees of many countries are multisectoral in principle but they do not appear to have met very often, and non-health ministries, with the occasional exception of education and defence, have rarely been involved in planning and implementing AIDS-related activities. Most sectors of government consider AIDS to be a health issue and are rarely motivated to get involved in HIV prevention.

> Some countries have now decided to vest responsibility for planning and coordinating AIDS activities in a central body, such as the ministry of planning, or a national commission. Uganda, for example, has established a National AIDS Commission...The New Commissions include all relevant ministries, as well as NGOs and the private sector. They have been supported by WHO, UNICEF, UNDP, the World Bank, and USAID, and imply a more traditional role for WHO as technical advisor to the Ministry of Health.[38]

UNAIDS

The Joint United Nations Programme on HIV/AIDS – UNAIDS – was established in 1994 by a resolution of the UN Economic and Security Council, and in January 1996 it became officially operational. UNAIDS combined WHO's programme with those of UNICEF, UNESCO, UNDP, ILO, United Nations Drug Control Programme (UNDCP), and the WB. Corresponding to UNAIDS and the new global multisectoral strategy, it was acknowledged that AIDS programmes must move beyond conventionally defined public health interventions. The role of the UNAIDS was conceived as one of the 'catalyst' or coordinator of action on AIDS rather than a direct funding or implementing agency. The five core functions of UNAIDS are: leadership and advocacy for effective action; strategic information to guide the efforts of partners; monitoring and evaluation of the epidemic and the response; civil society engagement and partnership development; and financial, technical, and political resource mobilization and tracking.[39] According to its Director, Dr Peter Piot, the reorganization of the Global Programme was meant to '...make UNAIDS a more efficient, client-friendly programme. UNAIDS hopes to be the catalyst of a new alliance of governments, intergovernmental organizations, community-based organizations (CBOs), groups of people living with HIV infection and AIDS, the private sector, and academic and research institutions – in essence, an informal global alliance bound by a common commitment to challenging AIDS'.[40] Today, its budget is $95 million and it has a staff of 139. It stated mandate:

> As the main advocate for global action on HIV/AIDS, UNAIDS leads, strengthens, and supports an expanded response aimed at preventing transmission of HIV, providing care and support, reducing the vulnerability of individuals and communities to HIV/AIDS and alleviating the impact of the epidemic.[41]

It was indeed the case that within the WHO there was a disjuncture between the general understanding of the global AIDS epidemic – as multidimensional and more than just a health issue – and its translation into policy. The solution to the weaknesses of global AIDS policy was to be found in a more integrated perspective; through proper expert knowledge, and the efficient and cost-effective implementation of a broader range of interventions to be implemented by a wider range of communities, NGO and private-sector partners. In engaging the range of UN agencies, each could bring its distinct focus of expertise to the global response; for example, the UNDP was the convening Agency on Governance and Development Planning responsible for coordinating and implementing a multisectoral response; United Nations Fund for Population Activities (UNFPA), the convening Agency on Young People and Condom Programming; UNICEF, on orphans and children affected by HIV/AIDS, and UNDCP, on addressing all aspects of the drug problem; ILO, on mobilizing workers and employers against HIV/AIDS and developing workplace standards and codes of practice; UNESCO, on appropriate education for prevention; and WHO, on strengthening the health sector response. The WB has its own Multi-country HIV/AIDS Project for Africa and the Caribbean (MAP) involving more than $1 billion, which receives advice from UNAIDS and its co-sponsors.[42]

In the 1990s, as it was becoming clearer that AIDS was having an impact in countries reaching far beyond family tragedy and strains on the health care sector, the most poorly articulated goal of UNAIDS was the mitigation of impacts of the epidemic – although this was to be up to 'communities'. Added to the list of strategies are programmes targeted at orphans such as school-fees relief, income generation, and support for extended families, as well as projects aimed at 'empowering' people and communities to cope better. With UNAIDS taking on the coordinating and catalyzing role, it was to be left up to the largely underfunded NGO sectors and local communities, with the assistance of the private sector, to implement programmes and projects at the community level to mitigate impacts. The lion's share of financial resources continues to be targeted at prevention programmes and medical interventions; data on resources being expended on this component is not even tracked, AIDS spending disaggregated into prevention, care, and research.[43] Barnett and Whiteside claim that despite the much broader perspective behind the formation of UNAIDS, and its efforts to include social and economic aspects in its work plans, the main focus has been on the clinical medical, and behavioural levels, with scant attention paid to country programmes, Ministries of Health and government policies, to the broader factors which contribute to the risk environment of AIDS.[44]

The community response

Across the political spectrum today, the community is invoked as the main actor in development; with NGOs increasingly viewed as the organizational mechanisms through which 'the community' can be empowered. The shift in expenditure from the state to NGOs in the past decade has been significant – USAID, for example, was channelling 87 per cent of its aid to Kenya, directly to NGOs and the private sector in 1995.[45] The shift stems in part from the failure of the state as an agent of development – by virtue of being 'not the state' NGOs are worthwhile vehicles for development assistance. NGOs mushroomed across the continent throughout the 1990s as a response to AIDS, assuming the delivery of many of the social services that have been abandoned by the state. The NGO sector has grown in both scale and diversity over the course of the AIDS pandemic.

Non-governmental Organization emerged essentially as emergency relief organizations in the aftermath of wars in Europe and Africa: Save the Children started in the 1920s, Foster Parents Plan after the Spanish Civil War, Care and Oxfam after Second World War and Médecins sans Frontières (MSF) after the Biafran war in Nigeria. Included under the umbrella term, NGO includes the 'super NGOs' with cross-national membership revenue-generation potential. The following revenues give some sense of the scale of activities: Care International had over $586 million in 1996; the Oxfam Network had a combined income of $350 million; and MSF had over $252 million the same year.[46] With the growth and consolidation of these super NGOs – the apparent globalizing of the NGO movement – some have taken on more of a policy dialogue and lobbying/advocacy role. Certain NGOs aligned with bilateral donors such as USAID have explicitly neoliberal agendas, while others, MSF, Oxfam, Human Rights Watch, for example, have been instrumental in focusing international attention on the disparity between North and South with regard to access to treatment, and have also worked in partnership with UNAIDS and other multilateral agencies. NGOs certainly do not share the same sets of values, and many can and do have a positive impact. Some NGOs have been at the forefront of the movement for global justice known somewhat inaccurately as the antiglobalization movement. Oxfam and Save the Children have spearheaded campaigns to cancel African debt and to promote human rights; in 2002, the Oxfam Network set off minor shock waves when they published a report on globalization entitled 'Rigged Rules and Double Standards: Trade, Globalization, and the Fight against Poverty', in which they called for a comprehensive review of existing trade regimes.[47] As mentioned in the previous chapter, international NGOs such as Amnesty International and Human Rights Watch have been central in focusing attention on the human rights violations that have increased as a result of the intensification of AIDS epidemics, such as property rights violations against AIDS widows and sexual violence against women, while MSF and Oxfam have taken on TRIPs and the WTO.

In response to SAPs and reductions in state expenditure on health, education, and rural development, the volume of donor support channelled through NGOs rose, mostly in the form of grants but increasingly by means of contracts.[48] The lines are increasingly blurred in the state–market–civil society nexus. Private corporations have been known to contract NGOs to provide services (to give an example, the large Canadian-based mining multinational, Barrick Gold, has been working 'in partnership' with Care Tanzania who received the sites and services contract for a mining resettlement project for the Bulyanhulu Mine in Tanzania); bilateral donors often carry out their development assistance policy through their own national NGOs working overseas (for example, USAID funding World Learning in Africa) and International NGOs are often the main sources of grants for local indigenous NGOs and grassroots organizations. The huge mushrooming of NGOs in Africa can be seen as problematic for a number of reasons. Julie Hearn and others have argued that the shift in funding to NGOs in Africa is part and parcel of the New Policy Agenda of neoliberalism – NGOs acting as a direct substitution for the state in service provision, and a counterweight to state power.[49] NGOs in effect reconfigure the relationship between the private and public, shifting the responsibility for social policy away from the state and towards the voluntary sector and the market. The state can ignore the plight of its citizens while NGOs compete for project funding. NGOs create new circuits of power and hierarchy in the societies within which they operate, and are not necessarily accountable to their local constituents but to those who control the purse strings. They often do not reach those most in need, and cannot act as a substitute for a minimum core of broadly accessible services provided by states. Ultimately, they leave unresolved the macrolevel economic and political forces that underpin local inequalities.

That being said, NGOs have been the main vehicles for the imple-mentation of the institutional response outside the orbit of basic biomedical interventions such as epidemiological surveillance. Included in the mix have been International NGOs with branches in SSA (among the most active are Save the Children, World Vision, Action Aid, African Medical and Research Foundation (AMREF), World Learning, MSF, Oxfam, CARE); indigenous NGOs have included churches and religious institutions, trade unions, cooperatives, and small community-based women's organizations. NGOs have been centrally involved in all aspects of the response to AIDS.

The initial approach of the GPA's first Director, Jonathan Mann, was strongly biomedical, but he challenged WHO protocol by trying to bring a broad range of civil society institutions around the table to help shape policy. Mann was considered a champion of human rights for the HIV/AIDS infected. And indeed, the issue of the relationship between HIV infection and poverty was aired early on in the epidemic, although in a way that was largely rhetorical. Mann created formal institutional space for AIDS Service Organizations (ASOs) within the GPA structure, initially promoting cooperation between the GPA and ASOs because of his belief that traditional Ministries of Health – the usual counterparts of WHO in member states – were not equipped to address the emerging pandemic alone.[50] In November 1988, a Draft Strategy for GPA–NGO Cooperation was circulated; in the same year, a special post of External Relations Officer for NGOs was created. The first conference on NGOs Working on AIDS was organized as a pre-conference to the Fifth International AIDS Conference in Montreal in 1989. On the top of the agenda of the over-100 NGOs was the proposed creation of an International Council of ASOs (ICASO); the next meeting in the following year would take up the question of formal representation in the GPA. At the Second International Conference on NGOs Working on AIDS, the problems with creating a collective NGO position on the international AIDS policy surfaced. The great diversity of groups working on the ground had difficulty formulating a common policy platform. The achievement of consensus was stymied not only by the individual grievances of different groups – gays, sex workers, Africans, women – with the status quo, but also with each other. Many coalitions of NGOs and ASOs working in the AIDS sector have since emerged, but many remain at arms length from the larger institutional actors.[51] ICASO has evolved into a network of networks with offices in Europe, Africa, Asia, North America, and Latin America, and is the most influential advisor of the NGO community to UNAIDS, with a mandate to ensure that those on the ground have a voice in global policy.

The activities of NGOs and grassroots organizations have spanned the breadth of AIDS interventions – prevention, treatment, advocacy, and mitigating impacts – although it is the latter, despite the high level of rhetoric devoted to the multisectoral response that remains largely marginalized and underfunded. In fact, most programmes have involved the design and delivery of education targeted at specific groups: women, men, youth, couples, prostitutes, miners, truckers, and children. 'Training of trainers' for peer education, advocacy for people with HIV/AIDS, improving access to experimental drug trials and health care, providing Zidovudine (AZT) to pregnant mothers to prevent perinatal transmission, and AIDS testing combined with pre- and post-test counselling are the main activities of NGOs. NGOs that have focused on home-based care are fewer and far between; the vast majority receiving no donor support and in some places, home-based care has contracted; in Zimbabwe, coverage dropped from 33 to 6 per cent between mid-1991 and 1995.[52] In a study of the largest community-care programmes in Zambia, actual coverage was only 7 per cent of the chronically ill population in the target area, and one of the main reasons given for such low coverage was the limited involvement of government in the provision of support for home-based care. Interventions in any case are often minimal, involving the distribution of palliative drugs (aspirin, antibiotics), food supplements, basic training for family members and community volunteers in caring for the sick, spiritual and emotional support, and mobilizing community support for practical household activities such as farming, chores, and assisting with funerals.

In effect, the response on the ground has made no difference to the vast majority of those affected by AIDS. There is a vacuum in research on specific NGOs, their scope, and geographic coverage, but it is a fair generalization to say that their activities have been concentrated in urban areas, and in areas of peace and stability. The WB states that programmes developed by NGOs have been slow to 'scale up' and that few resources have reached communities.[53] Estimates based on data from 2000 are that for SSA, HIV/AIDS spending amounted to 31 cents per person, and $8.16 per person living with HIV/AIDS, 'spending so miniscule as to leave millions without care and support' according to the International AIDS–Economics Network.[54]

But the new millennium has witnessed a commitment to finally respond to the African crisis. With echoes of AIDS as a famine and a security crisis, two high-profile institutional mechanisms were set up to deal with the impact of the crisis in Africa. The Global Fund to fight AIDS, TB, and Malaria (known as the Global AIDS and Health Fund) was established to mobilize billions of dollars from governments, corporations, charities, and individuals for the global pandemic, much of which would be disbursed to African countries. The projected need of the HIV infected in Africa alone was estimated in 2002 to amount to between $7 and $10 billion.[55] The money is to be targeted at prevention, basic medical care, and research. Contributions from Western nations have been paltry, totalling just over $2 billion over 5 years, with the Bill and Melinda Gates Foundation in 2002 matching Canada's contribution of $100 million. As of February 2003, *The Guardian Weekly* reported that it had raised in total by only 2.2 billion, and that there was 'no money left in the kitty' – the last funds having been disbursed among 60 countries.[56] Health Global Access Project (GAP) reported in June 2003 that the global fund needs $4 billion by the end of 2004 to cover the costs of the next three rounds of grants. George Bush announced $10 billion over the next 5 years for the US's bilateral AIDS programme in Africa and the Caribbean, of which only $1 billion is slated for the Global Fund. The programme is seen by some as a slush fund for US pharmaceutical companies, citing 'buy American' rules in USAID. Action Aid notes that one-third of the expenditure allocated to prevention is aimed at projects that promote abstinence, a moralistic approach proven largely unsuccessful. The bill also links AIDS expenditure with acceptance of US GM food relief by recipient countries.[57]

The Annapolis Declaration was issued in 1999 through UNAIDS, pledging to create an International Partnership against AIDS in Africa (IPAA). The partnership has been conceived as a broad coalition of actors that, under the leadership of African governments, seeks to curtail the spread of HIV, reduce its impact on human suffering, and halt the reversal of economic and social development in Africa. 'Through the combined efforts of the actors (African governments, United Nations Organizations, donors, the private sector and the community sector), the IPAA is stimulating political awareness, mobilizing additional resources and strengthening national prevention and control programmes,' according to UNAIDS.[58] In a document that maps out the emerging strategy of the partnership, the principles of African ownership and leadership at all levels are spelled out, as is the need for the active involvement of people living with AIDS (PLWAs) in the partnership's design, implementation, and evaluation. The vision, though, is provided a priori:

> Through collective efforts, promotion and protection of human rights and promotion of poverty alleviation, countries will: substantially reduce new infections; provide a continuum of care for those infected by HIV/AIDS; mobilize and support communities, NGOs and the private sector, and individuals to counteract the negative impact of the HIV/AIDS epidemic in Africa.[59]

In September 2000, the WB launched its MAP to make available US$500 million in funding to 'scale up' HIV/AIDS efforts through the International Partnership; providing direct support to community organizations, NGOs, and the private sector for local AIDS initiatives. The conditions established by MAP include the agreement by governments to use multiple implementation agencies, especially NGOs, and government commitment to channelling grant funds to communities, civil society, and the private sector.[60] NGOs, 'communities', and the private sector are again singled out as the main actors in the delivery of AIDS programmes. Carolyn Baylies was at the 11th International Conference on AIDS and STDs in Africa which was an occasion for discussion of the initiative as well as the WB's new plan for AIDS prevention in Africa. She states that while using the language of partnership, ownership, and participation and calling on African governments to take the initiative and contribute economically, they have been brought into the partnership after the fact. And it is unclear how 'communities' are to be brought in, and resources allocated.

> All the while, there are those in communities who absorb the damage AIDS inflicts and continue, amidst great personal hardship, to help and support one another and to engage in campaigns of protection – in solidarity with a global morality more imagined than real.[61]

The WB's MAP Generic Operations Manual, drafted in April 2002 with input from the Kenya National AIDS Council Secretariat and reviewed by officials of nine African country governments and specialized agencies and donors, elaborates channels and mechanisms for involving communities and 'civil society', and spells out the role of National AIDS Secretariats, health sectors, and decentralized public sector agencies. It is a dense document, and certainly warrants more detailed analysis than I provide here. With regard to the public health sector, the document states that a strong health system is the foundation for the success in the fight against AIDS, and calls for 'scaled-up' and 'aggressive' programmes in partnership with NGOs and the private sector.[62] But deliverables are vertical AIDS-specific programmes (scaling up surveillance, setting standards for care and voluntary testing and counselling, aggressive STD and TB programmes, coordinating condom procurement, scaling up treatment and care including home care, and so on). In the context of weak and underfunded health care systems with low service delivery and poor capacity, it seems that it would make more sense to include as part of its MAP substantial debt relief, a realignment of resources towards the social sector, and a general strengthening of public health care system capacity.

Only four pages of the 122 page document are devoted to 'mitigation' despite the acknowledgement of the 'huge scale of the problem',[63] and that the 'age-old social safety net for children' is unravelling. The mitigation response is articulated through the window of orphans as an example of critical mitigation needs, but states that 'mitigation analyses and efforts should be expanded to all sectors (with respect to human resources and planning issues), gender issues, legal frameworks (property rights, etc.) and expanded to elderly populations caring for grandchildren, among others'.[64] In a nutshell, individual empowerment solutions are proposed to 'stimulate and strengthen community-based responses'. The policies which must be designed to prevent families from sinking into deep poverty as a result of the diversion of labour to caring for the sick or AIDS deaths include income generation, small business cooperatives, vocational training, and microcredit, all, of course, building the ubiquitous 'social capital'. Six lines are devoted to food security – a list of 'bookmark questions' that individual countries will need to ask about training, costs, sources of support, and implementation in food security. And six questions are posed concerning the elements good practice, resources, training, costs, and implementation experience of household-income programmes for national AIDS programmes to consider.[65] Completely absent is any consideration of the broader macrocontext and policy environment which threatens family income and food security.

Indeed, the most cost-effective way to mitigate impacts certainly is to 'empower' local communities to do so for themselves. One of the most popular solutions to the devastation of the impact of AIDS has been the 'promise' of microcredit:

> The AIDS epidemic is decimating the face of Africa. It is killing whole generations of mothers and fathers leaving a sea of orphans in its wake. On a continent already plagued by poverty, disease and hunger, there is a light of hope. A candle burns in the lives of Africa's poorest people: the hope and opportunity of microcredit.[66]

Microcredit schemes targeting women have burgeoned since the 1997 Microcredit Summit – the first privately organized development summit sponsored by major banks and credit institutions. The Summit launched a nine-year campaign to reach 100 million of the poorest people – a 'network of networks' involving donors, microcredit practitioners, educational institutes, International Financial Institutions (IFIs), and NGOs. The campaign's executive committee is a mix of public and private sector bigwigs, including the President of CIDA, the CEO of Monsanto, the Director General of the ILO, and George Soros. In Africa, many organizations have signed on as members of one of the 15 Microcredit Summit Councils – the database lists 158 in Kenya, 93 in Uganda, 36 in Tanzania, and 54 in Zambia. Under the campaign umbrella, the African Micro-enterprise AIDS Initiative, launched in 1999 by the global NGO Opportunity International and modelled on the Grameen Bank model, has as its goal to 'prevent the spread of HIV/AIDS by empowering women in Africa'.[67] Through its seven African partners, it seeks to reach five million women between 1999 and 2009, as well as to provide 'an innovative and sustainable model and blueprint for other groups fighting AIDS on the continent'.

In some cases, credit cooperatives have improved the lives of the poor. But the almost messianic zeal surrounding microfinance obscures the fact that its impact is largely unknown. There is no linear relationship between microcredit assistance and poverty alleviation, and in cases of severe impoverishment, impact studies have illustrated that a significant minority of people become worse off due to business failure, losses, and further indebtedness. The poor are not a homogenous group, and evidence suggests that the upper- and middle-income sections within the poor respond better to such assistance. Poverty has multiple dimensions, and when the macrodynamics of markets remain untouched, giving a poor person a loan does not automatically lead to 'empowerment'. Microcredit perhaps represents the ultimate neoliberal panacea for poverty alleviation, devolving responsibility for securing economic opportunity to individuals acting as responsible agents of their own well-being.[68]

Women are the preferred targets of microcredit because of their responsibility for household well-being; the theory is that 'empowering women' brings a multiplier effect – improving their economic well-being will improve that of their children as well. Not only do women invest their income in ways that benefit all household members, they are also a good-credit risk, exhibiting very high levels of loan repayment. The thinking behind the African Micro-enterprise AIDS Initiative is that through the combination of loans and AIDS education, women will gain both the knowledge to protect themselves and the socio-economic independence.

> Opportunity International is able to increase cultural and economic power, and enhance personal dignity. In the beginning of the loan cycle, the potential applicant is assessed on the strength of her character. Because she lacks traditional collateral, the Trust Bank must decide if her loan will be cross-guaranteed solely on the basis of her personal integrity. Although this may seem a risky proposition, OI has found that this is the first step in building women's dignity. By providing a loan, the Trust Bank says, "We believe in you" and places a measure of responsibility on her shoulders. Because the money given is a loan and not a hand-out, the woman's sense of self-worth is further strengthened. As she continues to build community with other women who have cross guaranteed her loan, she finds herself in an accountable support network. The woman accepts the money and invests it in her own micro business. As she begins to experience newfound financial independence, her sense of self-worth and empowerment grows. She is no longer constrained by economic forces to participate in sexual relationships which are dangerous and degrading. With each loan she receives and repays, the woman becomes increasingly stable financially and better equipped to negotiate her roles within her community. Sexual encounters become a matter of choice instead of obligation or necessity.[69]

The programme also targets women who are widowed and infected, including the ones who have been deprived of assets through widowhood and unfavourable laws, who possess a large number of dependents and few marketable skills. Very little research has been done on these women and their experience with microcredit – women who are already overburdened, in poor health, and struggling in critical poverty to hold together their families. As a substitute for public investment in health and education, 'self-help' and individual empowerment, particularly for those who are experiencing significant hardship, reflects a double standard that would never be applied to the well-fed and well-heeled, who have designed these programmes.

What does 'women's empowerment' mean in this context? As women in communities are articulated as the solution to alleviating the socio-economic impacts of the epidemic, women's 'private' domestic labour has intensified. People within communities experience the impacts of AIDS differently, on the basis of economic and social status and gender relations. Women for the most part continue to shoulder the responsibility of feeding and caring for their families, while current processes of economic restructuring that contribute to the undermining health and the destruction of the social and economic fabric of communities continue under-analyzed and unabated. In addition to this role, they are to become micro-entrepreneurs, in what amounts to a never-ending spiral of downloading to the most vulnerable. For what purpose are women becoming 'empowered' under these schemes?

Private business has also been asked to take on a greater role in managing the epidemic, the main incentive, its own self-interest since AIDS is considered one of the 'defining global issues that will affect market development and the performance of individual companies over the next half century'.[70] In 1997, the Global Business Coalition on HIV/AIDS, 'a rapidly expanding alliance of international businesses dedicated to combating the AIDS epidemic through the business sector's unique skills and expertise' was formed.[71]

> Our mission is to increase significantly the number of companies committed to tackling AIDS, and to making business a valued partner in the global efforts against the epidemic. HIV/AIDS should be a *core business issue* for every company, particularly those with interests in heavily affected countries. With the support of global

leaders in government, business and civil society, the GBC promoted greater partnerships in the global response to HIV/AIDS, identifying new, innovative opportunities for the business sector to join the growing global movement against this terrible disease.[72]

In 2002, Anglo Gold reported that between 25 and 30 per cent of its entire southern African workforce were HIV infected, with impacts on the company's profitability and the broader community within which it operates, and threatening any potential expansion.[73] The company, along with Anglo-American Corporation, and De Beers extended ARV therapy to infected workers. Coca Cola, the largest single formal-sector employer in South Africa and a partner of UNAIDS, came under intense political pressure for providing treatment only to its white-collar employees, leaving behind bottlers and distributors, and reversed the decision in 2002. But while a number of high-profile corporations have made announcements about their commitment to their HIV-infected employees, this has been in the context of a more general shift of the burden of AIDS away from the private sector. Sydney Rosen and Jonathon Simon present anecdotal and survey evidence of widespread burden-shifting practices in Zimbabwe, Nigeria, Botswana, and South Africa. The authors claim that pre-employment screening to exclude the HIV infected from the workforce, smaller employee benefits, restructured employee contracts, outsourcing of low-skilled jobs, selective retrenchments, and changes in production technologies to substitute capital for labour has been used to reduce the share of the economic cost of HIV-positive individuals borne by the private sector.[74]

Today, with the vast private concentration of wealth, there seems to be no alternative to the corporate philanthropy of the super-wealthy, what amounts to a modern-day Robin Hood strategy. The increased role for corporate philanthropy is reflected in The Hope For African Children AIDS Initiative (HACI), launched through the Bill and Melinda Gates Foundation, which brings together CARE, Plan International, Save the Children, the Society of Women and AIDS in Africa, World Vision, and the World Conference on Religion and Peace, to provide care, services, and assistance to AIDS orphans in 13 African countries to date. The goals of the programme are to reduce stigma, to treat opportunistic infections of parents and provide them with better nutrition to extend the parent–child relation, to help families plan for their deaths by helping them appoint guardians, writing wills, and counselling, facilitating children's access to education and life skills and mobilizing community caregivers. The programme is both relevant and assists those most in need. The question is whether it would exist even without the philanthropy of Bill Gates. The Gates Foundation has distributed $3.2 billion since its founding, to health projects in the Third World – its influence rivalling that of the WHO and UNICEF. An amount of $126.5 million has been pledged to the International AIDS Vaccine Initiative with 80 per cent of its contributions being funnelled through public–private partnerships.[75] The super-rich wield tremendous power to shape the global health policy agenda, whether their specific initiatives are appropriate and welcome.

Conclusion

The political counterpart to the economic dimensions of global restructuring, the ideology of neoliberalism, is reflected in the response, by its focus on cost-effectiveness as a determining factor in deciding on priorities; on vertical AIDS-specific solutions to the detriment of broad-based strengthening of the social sectors; on individual 'empowerment'; and on solutions that place the burden of care and mitigation of impacts on individual households through mobilizing 'local resources'. One of the basic contradictions between the discourse on AIDS policy and the policy response is the neoliberal model within which control strategies are implemented. The factors that fuel the spread of HIV – the same factors that facilitate the spread of disease in general in the African context: shrinking rural subsistence economies; increased migration and urbanization; instability and civil war; and a decaying or non-existent social safety net, all linked to broader socio-economic and geopolitical forces – are not considered proper 'targets' for 'intervention'. In essence, policies and projects are designed to empower people to protect themselves or to cope better with the outcome of infection. The response to African AIDS is largely depoliticized to the extent that it fails to acknowledge the vested interests that underlie the current global order, an order that contributes to the pattern of spread of HIV and disease in general. At the same time, contained within the AIDS policy are a set of practices which place neoliberal 'self-help' and individual empowerment solutions on the shoulders of the poorest of the poor. All the while, treatment is not a basic human right, but a luxury for the few.

Notes

1. Peter Lawrence, ed., *World Recession and the Food Crisis in Africa* (London: James Currey, 1986) 1.
2. Diane Elson, *The Impact of Structural Adjustment on Women: Concepts and Issues*, Report of the Women in Development Programme of the Commonwealth Secretariat (May 1987): 4.
3. Giovanni A. Cornia, 'Adjustment Policies 1980–85: Effects on Child Welfare', *Adjustment with a Human Face Volume 1*, eds Cornia, Jolly and Stewart (Oxford: Clarendon Press, 1987).
4. See, for example, David Moore, 'Levelling the Playing Fields & Embedding Illusions: "Post-Conflict" Discourse & Neo-liberal "Development" in War-torn Africa', *Review of African Political Economy* 27.83 (2000): 11–28; and Bonnie Campbell, 'Governance, Institutional Reform & the State: International Financial Institutions & Political Transition in Africa', *Review of African Political Economy* 28.88 (2001): 155–76.
5. Gerry Helleiner, 'Marginalization and/or Participation: Africa in Today's Global Economy', *Canadian Journal of African Studies* 36.3 (2002): 532.
6. Carol Thompson, 'Regional Challenges to Globalization: Perspectives from Southern Africa', *New Political Economy* 5.1 (2002): 42.
7. See, for example, Jean-Francois Bayart, Stephen Ellis, and Beatrice Hibou, *The Criminalization of the State in Africa* (Oxford: James Currey, 1999); John Craig, 'Evaluating Privitisation in Zambia: A Tale of Two Processes', *Review of African Political Economy* 27.85 (2000): 357–66; Morris Szeftel, 'Editorial: Globalization and African Responses', *Review of African Political Economy* 27.85 (2000): 353–57; Bonny Ibhawoh, 'Structural Adjustment, Authoritarianism and Human Rights in Africa', *Comparative Studies of South Asia, Africa and the Middle East* XIX.1 (1999): 158–67.
8. Bayart, Ellis and Hibou, xiv.
9. Ibid., 5.
10. Jean-Francois Bayart, *The State in Africa: The Politics of the Belly* (London: Longman, 1993) 4.
11. UNDP, *UN Development Report 2003* (New York: Oxford University Press, 2003) 3.
12. UNDP, 37.
13. Jeffrey Harrod, 'United Nations Specialized Agencies: From Functionalist Intervention to International Cooperation?' *The UN Under Attack*, eds J. Harrod and N. Schrijver (New York: Gower Press, 1991) 137.
14. Arturo Escobar, *Encountering Development: The Making and Unmaking of the Third World* (New Jersey: Princeton University Press, 1995) 41.
15. H. K. Jacobson, 'WHO: Medicine, Regionalism and Managed Politics', *The Anatomy of Influence: Decision-Making in International Organizations*, eds Robert Cox and Harold K. Jacobson (New Haven: Yale University Press, 1973) 205.

16. WHO, *Evaluation of Health Care for All by the Year 2000* (Geneva: WHO, 1987).
17. David Werner, 'The Life and Death of PHC', *Third World Resurgence* 42–43 (1994): 11.
18. Werner, 12.
19. Ibid., 18.
20. Kenna Owoh, 'The World Bank Investing in Health: Is This All There Is?' Conference paper, Hofstra University Conference *The United Nations at 50* (15–18 Mar. 1995): 5.
21. Kelley Lee and Hilary Goodman, 'Global Policy Networks: The Propagation of Health Care Financing Reform Since the 1980s', *Health Policy in a Globalizing World*, eds Kelley Lee, Kent Buse, and Suzanne Fustukian (Cambridge: Cambridge University Press, 2002) 116.
22. Lee and Goodman, 112.
23. Ibid., 166.
24. Fiona Godlee, 'WHO in Retreat: Is It Losing Its Influence?' *British Medical Journal* 309.6967 (1994): 1491.
25. See Godlee 'WHO in retreat'; Fiona Godlee, 'WHO's Special Programmes: Undermining from above', *British Medical Journal* 310.6973 (1995): 178; Fiona Godlee, 'WHO reform and global health', *British Medical Journal* 314.7091 (1997): 1359.
26. Kent Buse and Gill Walt, 'Globalization and Multilateral Public–Private Health Partnerships: Issues for Health Policy', *Health Policy in a Globalizing World* (Cambridge: Cambridge University Press, 2002) 42.
27. Stephen Lewis, 'AIDS, Conflict, Poverty: The Challenge for Canada and the UN', *Canadian Development Report* (2000): 5.
28. Buse and Walt, 49.
29. Transnational Resource and Action Centre, *Tangled up in Blue: Corporate Partnerships at the United Nations* (Corporate Watch, Sept. 2002) 5.
30. Transnational Resource and Action Centre, 58.
31. WHO/GPA, *Report of the External Review of the World Health Organization Global Programme on AIDS* GPA/GMC (8) 92.4 (Geneva, Jan. 1997) 5.
32. Jonathan Mann, Daniel Tarantola, and Thomas Netters, eds, *AIDS in the World* (Cambridge: Harvard University Press, 1992) 297.
33. Leon Gordenker *et al.*, 'International Cooperation on AIDS: A Report on Research Findings', conference paper, 1994 Meeting of the International Studies Association (Washington, 1994) 19.
34. WHO/GPA, 7.
35. Tony Klouda, *AIDS in Africa Panel*, Annual Meeting of the African Studies Association (Toronto: Nov. 1994).
36. WHO/GPA, 5.
37. Ibid., 24.
38. Ibid., 18.
39. Joint Session of the EXEC Boards of UNDP/UNFPA, UNICEF and WFP, 'HIV/AIDS: Addressing the Recommendations of the UNAIDS Five Year Evaluation' (9 June 2003): 2.
40. Peter Piot, qtd in 'Update: UNAIDS Gets Swedish Support', *AIDS and Society* 6.4 (July–Aug. 1995): 9.

41. UNAIDS, 'About UNAIDS' (UNAIDS, 13 May 2002) (http://www.unaids.org/about/index.html).
42. UNAIDS, *UNAIDS Partnership*: *Working Together on AIDS* (Geneva: UNAIDS, May 2002).
43. See Priya Alagiri, Todd Summers, and Jennifer Kates, *Global Spending on HIV/AIDS in Resource-Poor Settings* (Henry J. Kaiser Family Foundation: July 2002).
44. T. Barnett and A. Whiteside, *AIDS in the Twenty-First Century*: *Disease and Globalization* (Basingstoke: Palgrave Macmillan, 2002) 73.
45. Julie Hearn, 'The NGO-isation of Kenyan Society: USAID and the Restructuring of Health Care', *Review of African Political Economy* 25.75 (Mar. 1998): 90–91.
46. Christopher Gombay, *Canadian Non-governmental Organizations and CIDA: Whither Canadian NGOs?* Paper prepared for the Canadian Council on Social Development (2002).
47. Gombay, 6–7.
48. Mark Robinson, 'Privatising the Voluntary Sector: NGOs as Public Service Contractors?' *NGOs, States and Donors: Too Close for Comfort?* eds David Hulme and Michael Edwards (New York: St Martin's Press, 1997) 61.
49. Julie Hearn, 89–101.
50. Peter Soderholm and Roger Coate, 'Institutionalized Chaos: AIDS, Environment and World Politics', conference paper, 34th Annual Meeting of the ISA (Mexico: Mar. 1993) 22.
51. Solderholm and Coate, 22–39.
52. Emmanuel Fru Nsutebu *et al.*, 'Scaling up HIV/AIDS and TB Home Based Care: Lessons from Zambia,' *Health Policy and Planning* 16.3 (2001): 250.
53. World Bank, 'About MAP' (http://www.worldbank.org/afr/aids/map.htm).
54. Steven Forsythe, ed., *State of the Art*: *AIDS and Economics* (International AIDS Economics Network, July 2002) 3–5.
55. N. K. Poku, 'The Global AIDS Fund: Context and Opportunity', *Third World Quarterly* 23.2 (Apr. 2002): 283–98.
56. Boseley, Sarah, 'UN AIDS Fund Empty as US Offers $15bn', *The Guardian Weekly* (6–12 Feb. 2003): 5.
57. Harinder Janjua, *The Best Chance We Have*: *The Global Fund to Fight AIDS, TB and Malaria* (Action Aid, 16 June 2003).
58. UNAIDS/Programme Coordinating Board (9)/00.4 (Geneva: UNAIDS, May 2000).
59. UNAIDS/Programme Coordinating Board, 4.
60. World Bank, 'About MAP'.
61. Carolyn Baylies, 'International Partnership in the Fight Against AIDS: Addressing Need and Redressing Injustice?' *Review of African Political Economy* 26.81 (1999): 388.
62. World Bank, *MAP Generic Operations Manual* (World Bank, Apr. 2002) 45.
63. World Bank *MAP*, 118.
64. Ibid., 118.
65. Ibid., 121.

66. Microcredit Summit Campaign, 'Microcredit Helps Ease the Burden of AIDS in Africa' (http://www.microcreditsummit.org /press/AIDS.htm).
67. Microcredit Summit Campaign, 'African Microenterprise AIDS Initiative', 1 (http://www.microcreditsummit.org/press/Africanmicro.htm).
68. Katharine N. Rankin, 'Governing Development: Neoliberalism, Microcredit and Rational Economic Woman', *Economy and Society* 30.1 (Feb. 2001): 18–37.
69. Microcredit Summit Campaign, 'African', 7.
70. B. Plumley, P. Bery, and C. Dadd, 'Beyond the Workplace: Business Participation in the Multi-sectoral Response to HIV/AIDS', conference paper, XIV International Conference on AIDS (Barcelona: July 2002) 2.
71. Global Business Coalition on HIV/AIDS (http://www.businessfightsaids. org).
72. Global Business Coalition on HIV/AIDS, 'What We Do' (http://www. businessfightsaids.org/about_what.asp).
73. Plumley *et al.*, 1.
74. Sydney Rosen and Jonathon Simon, 'Shifting the Burden: The Private Sector's Response to the AIDS Epidemic in Africa', *Bulletin of the World Health Organization* 81.2 (2003): 131.
75. Stephanie Strom, 'Gates Aims Billions to Attack Illnesses of World's Neediest', *New York Times* (13 July 2003).

3
The Other 'War on Drugs'

Perhaps no single issue has come to define the political activism of the global HIV/AIDS pandemic more than the issue of the glaring global inequality in access to life-saving treatment. As Laurie Garrett put it, 'HIV was, by the close of 1999, a lightning rod for protest against pharmaceutical companies, trade related intellectual property rights (TRIPS), and global inequalities in public health'.[1] The establishment of the WTO and its expansion of international trade law into the sphere of pharmaceutical research and development as codified in TRIPS has prompted international outrage, and intense public debate and protest. A global movement has evolved to secure access to AIDS drugs, led by MSF, Oxfam, Consumer Project on Technology (CPT), Treatment Action Group (TAG), Health Global Access Project (GAP), and Health Action International. At the same time, national coalitions have emerged in SSA, such as South Africa's Treatment Action campaign (TAC), the Kenya Coalition for Access to Essential Medicines, and the Uganda Coalition for Access to Essential Medicines. The movement has exposed the failure of current international trade law and the global market system for getting treatment to those who need it most; but pressure has also been directed towards governments for not providing life-saving drugs, particularly in the face of the recent price breaks negotiated between various countries and pharmaceutical suppliers. Access to HIV treatment has emerged as the 'vanguard struggle' to the extent that political mobilization of the global HIV/AIDS movement has focused first and foremost on the right to treatment.

The problem of access to ARVs in SSA is part of a deeper problem of the commodification of basic human necessities, a problem that has life-and-death implications for many people. These processes pre-date the WTO and TRIPS. But they have intensified with the increasing concentration of power and wealth in the hands of a few and the entrenchment of a set of beliefs and practices having no moral or empirical foundation about who the emerging global system should serve – global capital at the expense of securing basic human needs. The HIV/AIDS pandemic graphically illustrates not only the fallacy of the market mechanism as the most efficient, beneficent arbiter of wealth and life chances, but also the hypocrisy of those who stand behind the ideology of free markets while flexing their muscle in forums like the WTO to further deprive those existing on the margins of the purported benefits of globalization's spoils – increased growth and trade, and scientific and technological advancement.

Pharmaceutical research on HIV/AIDS has taken place in a context of increased commodification of knowledge production, diminished public funds for medical research, and the deepening of university–industry relations. Private sector funding has become more and more essential to public sector research in Canada, the US, and the UK, and as Moony states, 'it is clear now that at least in the US the private sector has a dominant influence over the direction of public research... corporations can skim off the cream of publicly funded research for their own private benefit'.[2] The independence of public sector agencies and universities to set priorities has been thrown into question as universities and publicly funded research institutes increasingly play the role of knowledge industry for the corporate sector. James Love of the Center for Study of Responsive Law has pointed out that two ARVs, AZT and didanosine (ddI) were developed by the US National Institutes of Health at the expense of taxpayers, yet have generated huge profits for the pharmaceutical companies which have produced and marketed them.[3]

In December 2000, less than one-tenth of one per cent of HIV-infected people were receiving ARV therapy in Africa,[4] the majority being wealthy urbanites, formal-sector workers covered by company insurance schemes, and a few lucky participants in the scattering of pilot projects that are in place across the sub-continent. The reasons are complex, but the monopoly that the pharmaceutical companies have in setting prices for their patent-protected ARVs is a major factor – even vastly discounted prices for a year's treatment are roughly equal to the annual per capita income in many African countries. But the question of access to drugs in Africa goes beyond a consideration of the deepening scope of international trade law to include intellectual property. Patents are only one part of the equation to the extent that even at prices that are a fraction of the market price, it is not clear how those most in need, particularly people living in rural areas, would be provided with treatment. In many regions, beleaguered health care systems are starved of human and financial resources and have a limited reach. As already mentioned, up to half the population in many countries have no access to even the most basic drugs to treat the most common infections.

One must also ask why it has taken almost 20 years into the epidemic to see a concerted effort to develop a vaccine. Certainly a factor is that the industry itself establishes research priorities. The focus of pharmaceutical research and development (R&D) has been on treatments that can be sold in consumer-driven western markets, and AIDS drugs have been no exception. Jon Cohen wrote in 2001 that 'the search for an AIDS vaccine still cries out for leadership and coordinated research'. There are, as Cohen and others claim, formidable scientific obstacles to the development of an AIDS vaccine.

> HIV evades the immune system by altering its own make-up almost every time it infects a cell. Although most of those genetic variants are defective and cannot themselves make new viruses, there are enough viable variants to give nightmares to vaccine developers who favour the antibody approach. A vaccine made from one strain of HIV could indeed trigger antibodies, but those antibodies would probably work only against a small proportion of the many extant strains of the virus now circulating around the world.[5]

The so-called 'second-generation' vaccines – ones that focus on stimulating cellular immunity rather than producing antibodies – have shown no signs of being able to halt HIV completely. The eventual solution may come from a combination of vaccines that stimulate both the cellular immunity and the production of neutralizing antibodies, but whether a vaccine will even be discovered is still not a sure bet.[6] But Cohen also attributes the slow movement of vaccine science to the fact that there has been 'deep denial' on the part of researchers, industry, and governments. The pharmaceutical industry has shown little interest in the field 'because making and marketing an AIDS vaccine is simply not an attractive commercial proposition'.[7] Vaccines are far less profitable than drugs. Patients might require three doses of a vaccination over a lifetime, whereas patients with chronic illnesses might need to purchase drugs regularly for many years, as is the case with ARVs. With almost 80 per cent of the pharmaceutical market based in North America, Europe, and Japan,[8] a geographic area constituting less than 5 per cent of new HIV infections, it does not make economic sense to focus on vaccine development for the poor country market.

A vaccine provides no solution to those already infected with HIV, but given that the vast majority of new infections are occurring in poor countries, it is crucial to eventually put an end to the pandemic. But for those who are dying today, treatment is the more important issue, rather than the medium- and long-term prospects of widespread vaccination. People live in the short term. This is perhaps the main reason why activists have mobilized around the issue of TRIPS and extending access to ARV therapy, while public pressure for vaccine research has been somewhat more muted.

The TRIPs debate

In 1994, the General Agreement on Tariffs and Trade (GATT) evolved into the WTO, an international organization made up of member states with a mandate to reduce trade barriers to goods and services and to mediate trade disputes between countries. The WTO sets out the legally binding ground rules for international trade. As of April 2003, the WTO had 146 members, including 31 from SSA. Low-income countries have to comply with the agreement until 2006. The stated goal of the WTO is 'to improve the welfare of the peoples of the member countries'. Clearly, for some constituencies in some countries welfare has improved, but the general consensus is that the African continent as a whole has been made worse off. As Joseph Stiglitz, retired Vice President of the WB, contends, the antiglobalization protests began at the WTO meetings because it was the most obvious symbol of the hypocrisy of the advanced capitalist countries.

> While these countries preached – and forced – the opening of the markets in the developing countries to their industrial products, they had continued to keep their markets closed to the products

of the developing countries, such as textiles and agriculture. While they preached that developing countries should not subsidize their industries, they continued to provide billions in subsidies to their own farmers, making it impossible for the developing countries to compete. While they preached the virtues of competitive markets, the United States was quick to push for global cartels in steel and aluminium when its domestic industries seemed threatened by imports. The United States pushed for liberalization of financial services, but resisted liberalization of the service sectors in which the developing countries have strength, construction and maritime services.[9]

The US also accused the South of 'piracy' during the GATT Uruguay negotiations, claiming that it was losing more than $2.5 billion a year in royalties from copied pharmaceuticals.[10] Before the 1994 trade negotiations, a number of developing countries provided only partial or no patent protection to the pharmaceutical sector, in part because, as Philippe Cullet explains, they held the view that health was a basic need and the pharmaceutical sector should hence be protected from full commercialization.[11] Generic pharmaceutical producers, through the process of reverse engineering, were able to supply cheaper drugs that competed in the market with their brand-name originals. The strengthening of intellectual property law through TRIPS undermined the ability of members of the WTO to manufacture generics that were still under patent protection in the West, while extending and consolidating the monopoly power of a handful of giant pharmaceutical manufacturers.[12]

In theory, all countries have a say in trade negotiations at the WTO, but in practice, the agenda has been set by informal meetings of the major trading powers – the US, the EU, Japan, and Canada.[13] According to Carlos Correa, 'so far, the development and application of GATT/WTO rules have been strongly influenced by specific industries and commercial interests as illustrated by the deep involvement of multinational firms and various industry coalitions in the process leading up to the adoption of the TRIPS agreement'.[14] It was primarily at the instigation of two US-based companies, Pfizer and IBM, that the Uruguay round took up the issue of Intellectual Property.[15] Most African countries do not have a trade office in Geneva, and cannot afford a permanent presence. Furthermore, those sitting at the table in WTO negotiations are trade ministers who tend not to represent the broad interests of their countries but the interests of their narrower business constituencies. The claim that the WTO is by nature democratic can also be challenged to the extent that it excludes the participation of a broader representation of interests in the drafting of trade law despite its profound impact on all sectors of society. Trade law can enhance or hinder the exercise of basic human rights, as the case of access to ARVs demonstrates. It was unthinkable in the mid-1990s that health and local sustainable development considerations should be raised in WTO forums.

According to the WTO, intellectual property (IP) rights are 'rights given to people over the creations of their minds. They usually give the creator an exclusive right over the use of his/her creation for a certain period of time'.[16] Included today in the list of 'creations of people's minds' are things such as umbilical cord cells, human cell lines, and various indigenous peoples' medicinal plants and foods.[17] The majority of patents, in fact, are held not by 'people' but by corporations, giving them exclusive rights to commercialization. The granting of these individual 'rights' does not recognize the fact that scientific knowledge is cumulative and that today's discoveries are based on the acquired knowledge of researchers of previous generations, including knowledge derived from public institutions and from outside the laboratory. In the case of plant-based pharmaceuticals, original knowledge of efficacy has often resided within indigenous communities which unfortunately do not possess neither the sophisticated sequencing technology required to 'prove' their discovery and apply for a patent, nor the legal and financial power to challenge the patent applications of industry. Equitable protection of the IP of Africa's local communities – the biological resources and indigenous knowledge of farmers, healers, and plant breeders – has proven to be a major challenge.

Mark Heywood explains that 'historically, the granting of a patent was a reward, bestowed by the state, to an inventor *in return* for making the invention available to the public'.[18] What TRIPS accomplished was in fact the opposite; by tying access to medicines more closely than to purchasing power, it effectively left out three quarters of the world's population.[19] They are in fact a deviation from the principle of free trade by offering exclusive rights to the 'inventor' to exploit the invention and to stop others from doing so. With regard to pharmaceuticals, there are four basic categories of patents: patents on the chemical compound, on the compositional use of the compound as a drug, on the specific way the drug is used, and on the manufacturing process.[20] Hence a single drug can have many different patents. Under TRIPS, patent holders have exclusive rights to their invention for a period of no less than 20 years, but in the case of multiple patents on a single drug, the period of exclusivity can extend well beyond the 20-year period.

Supporters of the current patent regime make the argument that current levels of patent protection are necessary for R&D and innovation. Without the promise of high profits on a few successful drugs or 'blockbusters', companies cannot continue in the business of high-risk, high-failure research. It is the case that the development of new drugs requires huge expenditures for R&D and clinical trials, which are greater than the costs of production. The past two decades, however, have seen very little in the way of therapeutic innovation. According to Ellen 't Hoen, in the period 1981–1998, an assessment of 1779 new drugs in France showed that only seven could be considered a real therapeutic breakthrough, and that most were slight modifications of existing drugs.[21] Critics have also raised the issue of the vast amounts of money spent on advertising and marketing. A study of drug industry data for the year 2000 undertaken by Alan Sager and Deborah Socolar, Directors of the Health Reform Program of the Boston University School of Public Health, revealed that brand-name drug makers in the US were employing 81 per cent more people in marketing than in research, a gap that is widening. Marketing staff jumped by 59 per cent between 1995 and 2000, while research staff declined slightly. 'Large drug makers spend just one-third to one-half as much annually on R&D as they spend on marketing, advertising, and administration.'[22] Furthermore, Terri Nderitu explains that surplus profits went to stockbrokers and promotion amounted to $10.8 billion in 1998 and $74.8 million to lobby government in 1997.[23] In the run-up to the 2002 US elections, the sector made over $19 million in political donations, 95 per cent to the Republicans.[24] Evidence seems to suggest that the prices set for drugs reflect less the actual costs of R&D or their active ingredients, and more the costs of lobbying, marketing, and advertising. It is also not clear why the pharmaceutical industry needed the extra protection granted through the TRIPS agreement. Robinson points out that pharmaceuticals have been rated either first or second in the list of the most profitable sectors for more than thirty of the past 40 years. 'Drug companies have surpassed almost all other Fortune 500 companies in profit rates, outperforming Standard and Poor's 500 Index by 90 per cent and averaging profits more than three times that of other industries in *Fortune*'s survey.'[25]

Clearly, the patent system has not resulted in private sector R&D for diseases that do not make a profit – in essence, the diseases of the poor. The reason why cutting-edge drugs to treat HIV/AIDS are available is because the disease was initially a disease of the West, and hence there remains a captive and profitable market for drugs. According to the UN Human Development Report 2003,

> The imbalance between scientific effort and social need can be measured by assessing the share of total spending on a disease relative to the global disease burden – about 1:20 for malaria, a disease that kills more than 1 million people a year and debilitates the productivity of millions more. Malaria is almost entirely concentrated in poor countries (99 percent of all cases) and remains the primary cause of death in many.[26]

Supporters of the TRIPS agreement with regard to pharmaceuticals also point out that it contains provisions to ensure access to essential drugs; that exceptions to protect public health are built into the agreement. In fact, a number of exceptions and qualifications exist which could be used to support national policy goals. Article 8 of the TRIPS agreement states that 'Members may, in formulating or amending their national laws and regulations, adopt measures necessary to protect public health and nutrition, and to promote the public interest in sectors of vital importance to their socio-economic and technological development, provided that such measures are consistent with the provisions of the agreement.'[27] Article 27.2 allows states to restrict patentability of inventions if they pose a threat to human life or health.[28] TRIPS does not remove from member states the right to decide on their own laws for introducing parallel imports – the practice of purchasing a branded drug from a country where the drug is cheaper, as prices can vary significantly from country to country. Countries can also grant compulsory licences for production within their borders, allowing them to develop a generic equivalent of a patented drug without the patent holder's authorization (but with royalties paid to the patent holder) in the case of a health emergency. Compulsory licensing, however, is feasible only for nations whose market is big enough to support the manufacture of drugs. For the smallest and poorest countries, it is meaningless unless they can grant a licence to a foreign manufacturer, an issue that TRIPS give no legal certainty. In practice, it has proven to be less than straightforward for African countries to invoke these options. When they have, they have been met with the threat of sanctions from the US and legal action from the pharmaceutical corporations.

'Local' standards of care in Africa

There is still fairly widespread acceptance amongst policy-makers and government leaders, despite mounting protest, that the provision of drugs beyond the most cost-effective palliative drugs, and drugs to treat opportunistic infections is a given in the African context. In SSA according to the UNAIDS, at the end of 2002, 4.2 million died of AIDS but only about 50,000 were getting treatment. The WHO Essential Drugs and Medicine Policy, a list which contains safe and effective treatments for infections and chronic diseases which affect the vast majority of the population, did not include ARVs until 2002 because they did not meet all four of the criteria for inclusion in the list – safety, affordability, necessity, efficacy – the criteria being 'an uncomfortable mix of the clinical and economic' in Grey and Smit's words.[29] AZT and nevirapine were listed, but only to prevent mother-to-child transmission. The 13th edition of the Essential Drugs List of April 2002 added twelve ARV drugs, perhaps an implicit acknowledgement that economic criteria should not determine whether a drug is 'essential' or not. At this point, its inclusion is largely symbolic. As the list correctly states:

> Adequate resources and specialist oversight are a prerequisite for the introduction of this class of drugs. The antiretroviral drugs do not cure the HIV infection; they only temporarily suppress viral replication and improve symptoms. They have various adverse effects and patients receiving these drugs require careful monitoring by adequately trained health professionals. For these reasons, continued rigorous promotion of measures to prevent new infections

is essential and the need for this has not been diminished in any way by the addition of antiretroviral drugs to the Model List. Adequate resources and trained professionals are a prerequisite for the introduction of this class of drugs.[30]

The conditions listed in the WHO Essential Drugs List required to introduce ARVs – specialist oversight by trained health professionals and careful monitoring – are indeed a struggle in most African contexts. But the pharmaceutical industry has used the issues of widespread poverty and poor health infrastructures as evidence that patents have little to do with low access to treatment in Africa, and to justify inaction in addressing the fundamental issues relating to drug pricing. Two papers in particular, 'Do Patents for Antiretroviral Drugs Constrain Access to Treatment in Africa?' and 'Facts and Figures on Patenting and Access in Africa', received wide circulation by the pharmaceutical industry as evidence that other barriers are far more significant than patents in explaining the lack of access to essential drugs.[31] In response, James Love and Michael Palmedo of CPT closely examined where patents in SSA were filed, and reported on emerging trends. They found a concentration of patents where both the patients and the incomes are concentrated, and hence do represent a barrier in access to treatment.[32] In October 2001, Oxfam, TAC, CPT, MSF, and Health GAP issued a joint statement on the 'Facts and Figures' paper, challenging what they called the 'false conclusions drawn from the data':

The NGOs agree with the special communication's claim that many barriers impede access to health care in Africa, and support their call for international financial aid to fund antiretroviral treatment. However, they believe that the data presented in the paper do not support the conclusions drawn, but actually shed light on the extent of patent barriers to treatment. In African countries, the most practical and sought after combinations include fixed dose medicines (2 drugs in one pill) and affordable non-nucleosides. The most popular combination of AZT/3TC is patented in 37 out of 53 countries and the only affordable non-nucleoside (nevirapine in generic form) is patented in 25 out of 53 countries.[33]

The drugs that could be the most promising in the African context – the fixed-dose, two-pill-a-day combination – were the most patent-protected. In response to rather intense public pressure, pharmaceutical companies have responded with a tiered policy, or equity pricing, negotiating, on a one-to-one or group basis, price breaks on specific pharmaceuticals with various African governments, and have increased their corporate philanthropy; donating drugs to specific pilots and supporting AIDS projects through public–private partnerships. The other side of the coin has been their collective effort, with the help of the US government and the WTO dispute mechanism, to pressure countries that have invoked the emergency provisions of TRIPS in order to provide cheaper drugs to their citizens. In 1997, the South African government adopted a Medicines and Related Substances Amendment Act, giving it authorization for both compulsory licensing and parallel importing. Through the office of the US Trade Representative (USTR), the 'virtual strong arm of the pharmaceutical industry',[34] the US responded with the threat of trade sanctions to defend the IP rights of US manufacturers. The *Multinational Monitor* quotes a February 1999 report from the State Department saying that all of the relevant agencies of the US government – the Departments of State and Commerce, the US Patent and Trademark Office, the Office of the USTR, the National Security Council, and the Office of the Vice President – were engaged in 'an assiduous, concerted campaign' to persuade the South African government to withdraw or modify the Act. The US government responded to the Medicines Act in May 1998 by placing South Africa on its 'Special 301' watch list, the part of US trade law that requires the USTR to identify countries that deny 'adequate protection' for IP rights or 'fair and equitable access' for US persons who rely on IP law,[35] while the world's major pharmaceutical corporations brought a lawsuit against the South African government in the Pretoria High Court. (At the same time, the US issued a complaint through the WTO against Brazil, protesting its law to allow the manufacture and use of generic ARVs to treat the poor.) A coalition of CSOs based both in the US and in South Africa mounted a campaign against the US and the pharmaceutical companies that significantly elevated the profile of the issue internationally. As a result of the intense public protest, in September 1999 the USTR and the South African government announced that the dispute was resolved, with the US government announcing that it would cease putting pressure on the South African government on issues of compulsory licensing and parallel imports.

Other countries have also been subject to pressure and bullying. The newspaper *The Monitor* in Kampala reported on 8 May 2003 that the National Drug Authority has licensed three Indian companies to supply cheap AIDS drugs to Uganda, including Cipla Ltd, but that patent law banning the importation of generics could keep the drugs from coming into the country. When Cipla first exported products containing lamivudine and AZT into Uganda, chemicals that are covered by patents in Uganda, Glaxo Wellcome responded with a letter to the company asking them to cease all infringing activity in Uganda, stating that the IP protection was critical to expanding the global response to HIV/AIDS, 'including ensuring sustainable public–private partnerships such as the UN-led, nationally driven Accelerating Access Initiative'.[36] The Uganda Access to Essential Medicines Coalition raised the point that countries like Uganda are not required to comply fully with TRIPS until 2006, and wonders why the government had issued patents on these drugs. Uganda and other African countries have but little choice to follow the will of the US and the EU with regard to patent law because of their extreme dependence on donor assistance. But it also is the case that those in political office who bow to US or donor pressure benefit personally.

Hence protest has focused not just on the pharmaceutical industry and US government, but also on African leaders and Ministries of Health. Heywood points out that the South African government was spending $4 billion on re-armament, despite no apparent need or threat from its neighbours, while it was simultaneously arguing that it lacked the resources to expand access to HIV/AIDS programmes.[37] In January 2000, TAC announced legal action against the South African government on its failure to provide mother-to-child prevention programmes, and through a well-orchestrated campaign had public support for such programmes to be reinstated. TAC has also raised the issue of President Mbeki's questioning of the science of AIDS and in August 2003 it declared that withholding of ARVs by the South African government amounts to a 'crime against humanity' and has called for a stepped-up campaign of civil disobedience.[38] Shortly after, the government announced that it would provide ARVs through the public health system, a clear victory for TAC and its allies. It is still to be seen how they plan to implement the programme.

There have been clear victories on the part of TAC and its civil society allies over extending treatment for PLWAs, but South Africa happens to be the exception to the rule on the continent. It is the one country where a dollar a day for ARVs might be feasible. It is exponentially the largest economy in the region with per capita health expenditure amounting to $663 in 2000 (both public and private) and 3.7 per cent of GDP; per capita public expenditure amounting to $108. This contrasts with per capita public expenditure of $18 in Zimbabwe, of $6 in Mozambique and Tanzania, and of $4 in Uganda.[39] These figures illustrate the profound differences between countries. Within countries, there are deep inequalities in access to basic services as well as essential medicines. The percentage of the population with access to essential, affordable drugs (*prior* to the introduction of ARVs on the Essential Drugs List) in Zimbabwe, Uganda, Mozambique, and Tanzania is as low as 50 per cent according to the 2003 UN Human Development Report. In Uganda, 82.2 per cent of the population still lives on under $1 a day.

Scaling up treatment

The response to the pressure to scale up AIDS treatment outside South Africa thus far has been a combination of joint UN/pharmaceutical industry pilot programmes and projects, as well as other types of partnerships between NGOs, governments, charities such as the Gates Foundation, and pharmaceutical companies. UNAIDS and its co-sponsors instigated the 'Accelerated Access Initiative' in partnership with the pharmaceutical companies. In May 2000, five pharmaceutical corporations, Boehringer Ingelheim, Bristol-Myers Squibb, Glaxo Wellcome, Merck, and F. Hoffman-LaRoche began discussions with UNAIDS, WHO, the WB, UNICEF, and UNFPA 'to explore practical and specific ways of working together more closely to accelerate access to HIV/AIDS related care and treatment in developing countries'.[40] They were joined a year later by Abbott Laboratories and Pfizer. The statement of intent of the joint initiative acknowledges the need for strong national leadership, strengthened national health capacity and secure distribution systems, the inclusion of a broad range of actors, as well as more money for projects and continued investment in R&D on the part of the pharmaceutical industry for medicines relevant to the non-western world. It also emphasizes the importance of the protection of IP rights 'in compliance with international agreements, since society depends on them to stimulate innovation'.[41]

In a progress report dated November 2001, expanded drug donations and significant price breaks on a range of HIV/AIDS medications in many SSA countries were documented, a process however, by their own admission, described as slow and resource intensive, since it largely involved pricing discussions between individual countries and suppliers.

Major philanthropic endeavours involving both technical assistance and product donations were also noted. Bristol Myers Squibb's programme 'Secure the Future: Care and Support for Children with HIV/AIDS' was characteristic of the approach. Working in South Africa, Namibia, Lesotho, Botswana, and Swaziland is a $100 million five-year programme of medical research assistance to local scientists, community outreach and education grants, as well as support training in home-based care, participatory AIDS education, and income generation. Other companies have formed their own partnerships to broaden access to therapy and assist in other areas such as counselling and testing and AIDS education. All companies have made commitments to preferential pricing and expanded R&D. Some have partnered with ministries of Health to provide specific drugs free of charge. In Botswana, the country where levels of infection are the highest with an estimated 36 per cent of the adult population being infected, a new project, the African Comprehensive HIV/AIDS Partnership (Achap), involves the government working with the Gates Foundation and the pharmaceutical firm Merck, each funding one-third of the $150 million five-year initiative. The total cost of the package of care per patient is $1000 per year.[42] Pilot programmes to administer doses of ARVs to pregnant women have also been scaled up and preventing mother-to-child transmission has become a major priority. Not to question the legitimacy of such programmes, but little attention has been paid to the HIV-infected mothers of these babies, which begs the question of who is to care for them once their mother dies a premature death. Women are asking for these programmes with the knowledge that it is not deemed cost-effective to extend treatment to them, reflecting once again their expendability and the invisibility of their caring labour. UNICEF, a key player in implementing programmes for the prevention of mother-to-child transmission (PMCT), has proposed PMCT Plus, an initiative to provide women and mothers with ongoing care that may include ARVs for the mother. So far, these programmes are thin on the ground.

Despite the noted 'scaling-up', a progress report on the UN–pharmaceutical company partnership acknowledged in 2001 that the impact of the programme had been marginal, particularly in SSA. Middle-income countries had benefited the most, especially from negotiated price reductions, 'given their lower incidence of HIV infection and higher per capita incomes'. 'Gifts' from the pharmaceutical corporations and pilot projects have reached, but a tiny section of the HIV infected. Limited infrastructure to get the drugs to people and limited funding in relation to the cost of drugs were cited as the two main constraints to increased access. The progress report suggests recommendations to addressing these constraints: a more regional perspective; increased participation of the private sector in the development of health care infrastructures; stronger research collaboration in setting an operational and clinical research agenda between the UN system and the pharmaceutical companies; and more support, including enhanced private sector support, for the Global AIDS and Health Fund.[43] At issue is the sustainability of an approach which continues to rely heavily on private donations and pilot projects, and on the chronically undersupported Global AIDS and Health Fund, which shows a deficit of 50 per cent for the third, October 2003 funding round.[44] The underlying problems that exacerbate unequal access to treatment remain untouched. The dominant approach is unquestioning of international trade law as it now stands, the reliance on the private sector for drugs R&D, and the systemic problem of chronic underfunding of public health care systems.

But the global movement has had some impact. Emerging from the WTO meetings in November 2001, the WTO Declaration on TRIPS and Health – the Doha Declaration – was an affirmation that governments can take all necessary measures to protect public health. Led by the Africa group, a block of over 70 low-income countries pushed the US, Canada, the EU, and Switzerland into signing the agreement, which strengthened the measures that countries can use to protect public health to the extent that the declaration states:

> that the TRIPS Agreement does not and should not prevent Members from taking measures to protect public health. Accordingly, while reiterating our commitment to the TRIPS Agreement, we affirm that the Agreement can and should be interpreted and implemented in a manner supportive of WTO Members' right to

protect public health and, in particular, to promote access to medicines for all.[45]

While some activist groups see the agreement as a victory, others are less optimistic, pointing out that all what the declaration does is to affirm what already exists in TRIPS. Oxfam, in an international press release dated on the day that the declaration was signed, gave the deal a '4 out of 10 score', saying that although it sends a strong message that people's health should override corporate interests, the cost of the declaration for developing country governments was their agreement to widen the next round of trade negotiations to include high-speed talks on investment, competition, and industrial tariffs. Michael Bailey, the Senior Policy Advisor for Oxfam International, pointed to the rich countries' refusal to halt agricultural dumping or to free up its markets to exports from the LDCs, while pushing them to unconditionally open up their markets. 'These stark examples of double standards and hypocrisy indicate that the so-called "development round" touted by European governments has been buried in the Doha sand.'[46] The declaration also left unaddressed the issue of the importation of generics from countries like Brazil and India, which have pharmaceutical manufacturing capacity, to poor countries without that capacity or a sufficient local market to make production financially feasible. A promise was made to find an expeditious solution to the production-for-export issue, but it is yet to be found.

It also is the case today that health and the market are no longer considered in isolation – as a recent joint study by the WTO Secretariat and the WHO attests. *WTO Agreements and Public Health*, published in 2002, focuses on the main agreements of the WTO that have a direct bearing on public health – in addition to TRIPS, Technical Barriers to Trade, Sanitary and Phytosanitary Measures, and Trade in Services. Not surprisingly, the report is consistent with the view that the current IP law poses no direct threat to human health and, more generally, that a liberal international trade regime is beneficial to human health.

Trade liberalization can affect health in multiple ways. Sometimes the impact is direct and the effect is obvious, as when a disease crosses a border together with a traded good. Other times the effects of trade liberalization are more indirect. For example, reducing tariffs may lead to lower process for medical equipment and health related products; changing international rules concerning patent protection may affect the prices of medicines and vaccines. Important also, there is the link between freer trade and economic growth, which can lead to reduced poverty and higher standards of living, including better health.[47]

Written 'to enable both trade and health officials to better understand and monitor the effects of the linkages between trade and health policies', the report predictably reiterates the safeguards to protect health found in TRIPS and the Doha Declaration. It also deliberately omits a meaningful discussion of the relationship between trade and household food security 'because of its complexity'. There is an acknowledgement that malnutrition and undernutrition are responsible for about one-third of the disease burden in SSA, and as the report states: 'the great majority of the burden of disease associated with under-nutrition arises from chronic malnutrition as a result of *household* food insecurity'. Yet the report chooses to focus only on national food security, predictably stating that agricultural trade liberalization helps to improve export growth, 'thus providing more foreign exchange with which to import essential imports'.[48]

Conclusion: health and international trade law

Why do we have this problem? Is it because Jean-Paul Garnier, the CEO of Glaxo Smith Kline is a wicked man? No, the problem is with the commodification and privatization of medicine and with the evolution of something that for many people is essential to human life as water into something that makes profits for shareholders in countries in the first world. And this is made possible by the silent, but very deliberate, shifting of certain 'rights' away from the values that inspired them. Patent or 'intellectual property' rights are a case in point.[49]

In our increasingly globalized world, international trade law has emerged as a means of regulating finance, commodity, and information flows. The formulation of trade law has, up to now, been largely controlled by the representatives of capital, and has principally benefited corporate interests. The function of the law should be to facilitate the exercise of the rights of all of the community; to this extent, the basis and the test of justice and law is for human development.[50] It is not sufficient that trade law or 'rights' take into account human health – should the law itself operate in the service of the exercise of basic human rights, including health?

Most activists are not calling for abandonment of intellectual property regime altogether, but as 't Hoen asks: 'should the industrial agenda be set by industry alone? The present situation calls for an international approach to essential medical research and development to ensure that the vast amount of financial resources used for new drug development will lead to the production of products that address real health needs'.[51] One can go further and see that the right to access to essential medicines cannot be separated from a range of other rights – the right to food, shelter, security, knowledge, work, freedom of conscience, expression, association, self-determination. All humans have both physiological needs and purely human needs. The global distribution of resources for the exercise of these rights varies greatly, but is increasingly dependent on global laws and policies. As Cullet explains:

> From a broader perspective, even if deviation from TRIPS is allowed as an exception in the case of some health emergencies, this remains an unsatisfactory response from the perspective of human rights. It is not possible to distinguish the realization of the right to health from the eradication of poverty in general or the realization of the right to food and water. If exceptions are warranted in the case of health, they should be extended to all sectors related to the fulfilment of basic needs.[52]

Global activism surrounding TRIPS and the issue of access to treatment has accomplished much; it has heightened international attention paid to the relationship between trade law, and access to medicine and the huge disparities in access, and it has contributed to broader initiatives such as the Drugs for Neglected Diseases Initiative spearheaded by MSF and the International AIDS Vaccine Initiative, a global partnership of 'direct, goal-oriented research' to develop and distribute AIDS vaccines. It has tilted global opinion towards the view that the development of medicines cannot be left to the market place. But access to drugs is just one piece of a far more complex puzzle. The global neoliberal agenda, which includes the deepening commodification of life's necessities as codified in the WTO legislation, conditions the distribution of disease and the exercise of basic human rights essential to human health. Broadening and deepening the struggle to include a focus on the more complex aspects of the relationship between global trade and the right to health is just beginning.

Notes

1. Laurie Garrett, *Betrayal of Trust* (New York: Hyperion, 2000) 578.
2. Pat Roy Mooney, 'The Parts of Life: Agricultural Biodiversity, Indigenous Knowledge, and the Role of the Third System', *Development Dialogue*, Special Issue 1–2 (1996): 140.
3. Robert Weissman, 'Aids Drugs for Africa', *Multinational Monitor* 20.9 (1999): 7.
4. Terry Nderitu, 'Balancing Pills and Patents: Intellectual Property and the HIV/AIDS Crisis', *E-Law – Murdoch U Electronic Journal of Law* 8.3 (2001): 1 (http://www.murdoch.edu.au/elaw/issues/v8n3/nderitu83.html).
5. Jon Cohen, 'Deep Denial', *The Sciences* 4.1 (Jan.–Feb. 2001): 22.
6. Erika Check, 'AIDS Vaccines: Back to Plan A', *Nature* 423 (2003): 912–14.
7. Cohen, 22.
8. Mark Harrington, 'Brazil: What Went Right? The Global Access to Treatment and the Issue of Compulsory Licensing', conference paper, 10th National Meeting of People Living with HIV and AIDS (Rio de Janiero, Brazil, 3 Nov. 2000) 3.
9. Joseph E. Stiglitz, *Globalization and Its Discontents* (New York: W. W. Norton, 2002) 245.
10. Mooney, 137.
11. Philippe Cullet, 'Patents and Medicines: The Relationship between TRIPS and the Human Right to Health', *International Affairs* 79.1 (2003): 141.
12. Mark Heywood, 'Drug Access, Patents and Global health: "Chaffed and Waxed Sufficient"', *Third World Quarterly* 23.2 (2002): 225.
13. Peter Singer, *One World: The Ethics of Globalization* (New Haven: Yale University Press, 2002) 76.
14. Carlos M. Correa, 'Implementing National Public Health Policies in the Framework of WTO Agreements', *Journal of World Trade* 34.5 (2000): 112.
15. Heywood, 224.
16. WHO, 'What are "intellectual property rights"?' *Frequently Asked Questions about TRIPS* (http://www.wto.org/english/tratop_e/trips_e/tripfq_e.htm# WhatAre).
17. For a list of the 'World's 20 most outrageous patents', see Mooney, 150–54.
18. Heywood, 223.
19. Ibid., 226.
20. J. Robinson, *Prescription Games* (Toronto: McClelland and Stewart, 2001) 7.

21. Ellen 't Hoen, 'Globalization and Equitable Access to Essential Drugs', *Third World Network* (Aug.–Sept. 2000): 3 (http://www.twnside.org.sg/title/twr120c.htm).
22. Alan Sager and Deborah Socolar, 'Drug Industry Marketing Staff Soars While Research Staffing Stagnates', *RxPolicy* (6 Dec. 2001) (http://rxpolicy.com/studies/bu-rxpromotion-v-randd.pdf).
23. Nderitu, 8.
24. Sarah Boseley, 'UN AIDS Fund Empty as US Offers $15bn', *The Guardian Weekly* (6–12 Feb. 2003) 5.
25. Robinson, 2.
26. UNDP, *Human Development Report 2003*: *Millennium Development Goals*: *A Compact Among Nations to End Human Poverty* (Oxford: Oxford University Press, 2003) 158 (http://www.undp.org/hdr2003/).
27. Qtd in Correa, 107.
28. Cullet, 145.
29. Andy Gray and Jenni Smit, 'Improving Access to HIV-related Drugs in South Africa: A Case of Colliding Interests', *Review of African Political Economy* 28.86 (Dec. 2000): 584.
30. WHO Model List 13th Edition (WHO, Apr. 2003) (http://www.who.int/medicines/organization/par/edl/expcom13/eml13_en.pdf.).
31. Amir Attaran and Lee Gillespie White, 'Do Patents for Antiretroviral Drugs Constrain Access to Treatment in Africa', *Journal of the American Medical Association* 286(2001): 1886–92 and Tom Bombelles, 'Facts and Figures on Patenting and Access in Africa', conference paper, American Society of Law, Medicine and Ethics Conference (2001).
32. James Love with Michael Palmedo, 'Sub-Saharan African Patents by Population and Income: Draft', Consumer Project on Technology (6 Oct. 2001).
33. Médecins Sans Frontières, 'Patents Do Matter in Africa According to NGOs: Joint Statement by Oxfam, Treatment Action Campaign, Consumer Project on Technology (CPT), Médecins Sans Frontières (MSF) and Health GAP', press release (MSF, 17 Oct. 2001) (http://www.accessmed-msf.org/prod/publications.asp?scntid = 171020011428553&contenttype = PARA&).
34. Weissman, 6.
35. 'Under Special 301, countries that have the most egregious acts, policies or practices, or whose acts, policies or practices have the greatest adverse impact (actual or potential) on relevant US products and are not engaged in good faith negotiations to address these problems must be identified as "priority foreign countries". If so identified, the country could face bilateral US trade sanctions if changes are not made that address US concerns.' Warner Rose, 'The US Special 301 Process', *US Department of State: International Information Program* (http://USinfo.state.gov/products/pubs/intelprp/301.htm).
36. Letter from Glaxo Wellcome to CILPA on Importation of Duovir into Uganda (20 Nov. 2000).
37. Heywood, 220.
38. Reported on BBC International News (4 Aug. 2003).

39. All figures are for 2000, from WHO Selected Health Indicators.
40. UNAIDS *et al.*, 'Accelerating Access to HIV/AIDS Care and Treatment in Developing Countries: A Joint Statement of Intent' (UNAIDS, 8 May 2000).
41. UNAIDS *et al.*, 1.
42. Jo Revill, 'How Africa can Win the Battle against AIDS,' *Guardian Weekly* (31 July–6 Aug. 2003).
43. UNAIDS *et al.*, 20–22.
44. MSF Campaign for Access to Essential Medicines, 'AIDS Treatment Scale-Up Efforts Threatened: Donor Countries Fail to Fill the Funding Gap' (16 July 2003).
45. WTO, 'Declaration on the TRIPS Agreement and Public Health,' WTO Ministerial Conference 4th session (Doha: 9–14 Nov. 2001) WT/MIN(01)/DEC/W/2.
46. Oxfam International, 'Final Doha Declaration: Victory on Public Health but Few Other Gains for People in Poverty', press release (Oxfam, 14 Nov. 2001).
47. WHO/WTO, *WTO Agreements and Public Health* (WTO Secretariat, 2002) 23.
48. WHO/WTO 125–28.
49. Heywood, 223.
50. See John O'Manique, *The Origins of Justice: The Evolution of Morality, Human Rights and Law* (Philadelphia: University of Pennsylvania Press, 2003) 112–31.
51. 't Hoen, 3.
52. Cullet, 155.

4
Why Africa? Uganda's Epidemic in Historical Perspective

In the pages that follow, I present an analysis of the historical foundations of Uganda's AIDS epidemic. The purpose is twofold: first, to illuminate the features of the region's economic and political development that help to explain the contemporary spread of HIV; and second, to provide the general historical context of the institutional response during the past two decades. I want to tease out of colonial history the factors that have contributed to high levels of infection, and to today's local politics of survival in Uganda. The three factors that I focus on are colonial land policies, labour policies, and social policy as administered through missionaries. During the colonial period we see in Uganda the introduction of the system of migrant labour, and the economic development of some regions at the expense of others, causing significant societal disruption at multiple levels – from the personal to the regional. These processes further eroded women's position within their communities and precipitated the breakdown of the extended family system in some regions – the very system that is the supposed backbone of the contemporary community response to HIV/AIDS. The immediate post-colonial period further entrenched the conditions that led to Uganda's high levels of HIV spread during the 1980s.

Exploring the historical roots of the AIDS crisis in Uganda helps to clarify the links between the broader social and economic organization of society and disease spread. The factors fostering HIV spread vary between different regions in SSA, but despite the specifics, in all cases gender relations are key – not simply as relations between individual men and women, but as relations of inequality encoded in land and labour policies, and in access to power and resources in local communities. Within the East Africa Protectorate, African women were singled out by colonial officials as one of the main problems; displaying high levels of 'promiscuity' and STDs, which in turn contributed to low birth rates and high infant mortality. But these features of the early colonial period reflected, according to Megan Vaughan, 'a number of intertwined problems, including changes in property rights, in rights to labour, and relations between generations... the real issue... was that with far-reaching changes taking place in economic relations, enormous strains were placed on both gender and generational relations'.[1]

What were those changes? I want to suggest that the transformations in gender, generational, and familial relations were related to the disruptions in the rights and obligations of men and women – both social and economic – within the kin corporate societies that came under the control of indirect rule in the region that is today Uganda. I do not wish to paint a romantic picture of a rosy past – there were serious intra- and intersocietal tensions in the region before the British arrived. In Bayart's words, 'Africa did not have to wait for the arrival of the Europeans before it witnessed the disappearance or weakening of its communities through conquest, economic decline, cultural assimilation, demographic weakening or ecological disaster.'[2] Nevertheless, the dislocations that marked the onset of colonial rule were radical and sweeping and did overthrow a more stable order.

Colonial rule was formally codified in the Buganda Agreement of 1900 which established the pattern of relations with the precolonial state of Buganda, and in turn provided the blueprint for the integration of other local societies into the protectorate of Uganda. The British employed the Bagandans – the most powerful and centralized state of the Great Lakes region, Buganda – as agents of their imperialism, a policy commonly referred to as 'Buganda sub-imperialism'. The Baganda gained in wealth and power through its role as agents of the British over the non-Baganda.[3] Buganda's status as a mini-state within the protectorate served to foster division and disunity in the colony as a whole. Underlying the Buganda Agreement was the view that the long-run interests of Britain would be most effectively served through the creation of a 'landed gentry' capable of acting as an intermediary between the British and the Buganda peasantry. This was accomplished by formalizing land tenure systems with origins in the precolonial system of land tenure, but with greatly expanded discretionary land distribution being removed from the Kabaka – the King – and transferred to the Lukiko – the Parliament or General Assembly of Buganda. Under the terms of the Buganda Agreement, 1003 square miles of land were allotted to the king and to the big chiefs while an additional 8000 square miles were distributed to approximately 1000 chiefs and landowners at the discretion of the Lukiko.[4] This land – which came to be called mailo land – was enshrined as was freehold (for churches and schools); leasehold (alienated to the protectorate government); and customary tenure. As a result of the agreement, the crown came to possess about three-fifths of the area of Buganda.[5] So long as the Kabaka and the chiefs cooperated with the protectorate government, the structure of the Buganda state would be maintained and the Kabaka would remain its native ruler. Similar agreements were signed with other kingdoms falling under protectorate control, Ankole, Bunyoro, and Toro, but according to Mutibwa, they were inferior to the one between the British and Bugandans.[6]

According to A. B. Mukwaya, the framers of the Uganda Agreement assumed that they were codifying in permanent form existing rights and privileges, whereas in practice the rights conferred on individuals who constituted a fundamental change in the traditional system.[7] The main provisions of the law stipulated that an individual could own up to 30 square miles, and could transfer the land by sale, gift, or will; and only where a will was not left, would succession be determined by customary rules. Customary rights to the use of roads, running waters, and springs would be preserved.[8] Peasants continued to assume the same relations with the mailo owners as they had under the old type of kinship or political chiefs, and mailo owners received the same type of services and dues from their tenants as previously expected. With cotton production, mailo owners demanded either use of customary labour or a portion of the cotton or cash equivalent.

The law made no distinction between men and women as mailo owners, although very few women were allotted any land; only notable members of the aristocracy. The registration of titles showed that in 1920, 3.5 per cent of land was held by women; this gradually increased to 15.3 per cent by 1950.[9] It was legal for women to inherit land, but 'traditional' customs of inheritance were maintained whereby a man would be succeeded by one of his male clan relations. If a man left behind no written will, a wife would have no right to her husband's landholding or the products of her labour. This was also the case for peasants. Once a man died, or gave up rights to customary tenancy, his wife had no legal rights of use to the land or to her production. The land and her produce would revert back to the mailo owner.

With the privatization and individualization of land largely in male hands, women's rights as sister within her natal kin group were undermined. This was a change from pre-colonial land tenure relations, in which women maintained certain rights to land and resources on the basis of their status as daughter or sister. Previously, land had not been privately owned by men but the kin corporation was the land-holding unit. The same was true for men's and women's sexuality. As Nakanyike Musisi puts it previously, 'women did not own their egg, and men did not own their sperm; sex was a resource to be deployed by the lineage'.[10] The colonial move to the private ownership of land resulted in a parallel move in which men could own, individually, female sexuality and reproductive labour. In Buganda this was reflected, for example, in some women taking their husband's last names for the first time, a change from the previous practice of maintaining their last name which at birth was given to them in honour of a clansmember.

The Buganda Agreement also codified the specific rights and obligations of the respective communities, the methods and monetary limits of taxation, and the institutional character of native authorities. It also spelled out the regime of extra-economic coercion, in Mahmood Mamdani's words, 'the compulsion by which free peasants with customary access to land may otherwise be conscripted, forced to labour, or to cultivate – that makes intelligible the powers chiefs wielded over peasants'.[11] While civil law evolved to regulate market relations, the customary power of appointed 'chiefs' was located at the axis of market and non-market relations, the link mediated through the extra-economic coercion of the peasantry.[12] Mamdani argues that British rule in Uganda – as with European rule in Africa more generally – came to be defined by 'a single-minded overriding emphasis on the customary'.[13] Indirect rule was not simply the continuation of indigenous forms of governance, but a recapitulation of custom and tradition based principally on the privileging of the institution of chiefship, an argument articulated a decade earlier by such scholars and Martin Chanock, and Hay and Wright.[14] Chanock suggests that customary law under the British represented a transformation of African institutions rather than a continuity; the ideology of 'tradition' and 'custom' used to justify what were, in effect, changes in the social and legal order underlying colonial exploitation. Mamdani describes the 'bifurcated' state as encompassing two forms of power under a hegemonic authority, civil and customary, with civil power reserved for the urban areas and non-African population, and 'customary' consolidating the non-customary power of colonial chiefs, '... enfor[ing] as custom rules and regulations that were hardly customary, such as those arising from a newly expanding market economy'.[15] Chiefs were answerable not to their communities, but to the British. In the societies of the north and east, where there was no tribal leadership on which to reconstitute relations of governance, chiefs were imposed from outside and new boundaries drawn up. This policy had devastating consequences particularly for the pastoral communities in the north, resulting in dramatic losses of pasture and livestock, and ecological decline.[16] Internal boundaries were also redrawn to ensure that each 'tribe' stayed put in their own county, as a means of facilitating the collection of taxes and maintaining 'law and order'. Resistance and survival strategies often degenerated into widespread violence and terror.

The unequal and uneven impact of colonialism

The first two decades of colonial rule were characterized by the establishment of commodity production in the southern regions of Buganda and Busoga, where coffee, rubber, cocoa, and to a lesser degree, flax, sugar, and tea were produced. But the most important crop was cotton, of very high quality, which was the ideal raw material for British textile production. Cotton production was dependent on cultivation by thousands of African smallholders. Cash cropping was carried out alongside subsistence production on plots averaging from five to ten acres per family.[17] In the cotton sector, the African smallholder system of production accounted for between 75 and 85 per cent of GDP during 1918–1919; by contrast, the plantation sector accounted for only 3 to 5 per cent of GDP.[18] However small, plantation agriculture was considered an important component of the colonial economy. The two systems were at odds with each other to the extent that the European plantation system was dependent upon the alienation of large tracts of prime agricultural land and the deployment of large numbers of semi- and unskilled African labourers. But the peasant sector also deployed migrant labour. Labour was also needed for the ginning and transporting of cotton.

Temporary migration from peripheral areas into the economic heartland of the country was achieved through the deliberate division of the country into producing and non-producing areas, with the north initially being the main labour-supply area. This policy served the colonialists' narrow purpose of ensuring that there was enough labour for production flowing into Buganda and Busoga. This policy was slightly adjusted in the 1920s when the colonial government began to encourage the cultivation of economic crops in outlying districts. At this point, Uganda began to receive substantial amounts of cheap labour from the neighbouring states of Rwanda and Burundi. Nonetheless cash cropping remained marginal to the economy in the north; the general pattern under which the people from the north provided labour to the commodity-producing areas, and soldiers for the army became institutionalized in the first two decades of colonial rule.

A hut tax of three rupees per annum imposed under the terms of the Buganda Agreement initially compelled a great increase in the number of people seeking paid employment, thereby providing the colonial government with a solution to the problem of how to create a 'voluntary' labour force. In 1905, a poll tax of two rupees was added, the result being that a local labour supply sufficient to meet the requirements of the government and the private sector emerged in Buganda.[19] The initial supply of labour had diminished by 1908 however, when peasants discovered that it was easier to obtain money for taxes and imported goods by engaging in the cultivation of cotton.

The widespread trend towards the decline of women's status in SSA as a consequence of the introduction of colonial policies in general is well documented, which is not to say that there were some instances in which women appeared to maintain or improve their status.[20] An objective of colonial policy was the exploitation of both sexes, which necessarily had a deep effect on gender relations. Referring more generally to the African colonial experience, Mamdani points to the contradictory effects of the consolidation of chiefly power over previously autonomous social domains such as gender associations, age sets, and the household:

When it came to conflict-producing and tension-ridden relation-ships, freedom for one could only be at the expense of another. This was often the case with the marriage bond between male migrants on the move and female agriculturalists bound to village communities under the grip of a chief. As migrants appealed to tradition, chiefs often...imposed punishments for adultery and enforced paternal control over marriage. In migrant labour zones, women could and did turn into cash crop producing peasants, but their workload often increased alongside diminishing freedoms and increased compulsions.[21]

The historical record has very little to say about the changes in rela-tions between sexes accompanying changes to land tenure, the migrant labour system, and the transformation of production rela-tions. Evidence suggests that certain groups of women fared better than others under the changes introduced by the colonial adminis-tration – elite women in Buganda, for example, who were given legal title to land. In matters such as slavery, polygamy, and bride price, Victorian notions of right and wrong played a part in setting the practical limits to customary law. However, they were subordinate to political considerations, and therefore always negotiable.[22] In terms of changes in land tenure, women often stood out as victims of customary claims to the extent that the private male ownership of land rendered their customary rights to usufruct tenuous. Women's position as reproducer of the lineage came under stress as kinship ties became less important with the growth of the wage economy and the migrant labour system. Women's production for subsistence was intensified in the absence of males. At the same time, many women were drawn into cash crop production and according to a patriarchal notion of 'tradition', many women had no control of the cash proceeds of their labour.

The 'labour question', women's role in production, was indeed a prime concern of the colonial administration. As C. W. Hattersly, an official of the protectorate government, remarked in 1908,

The question of labour is at the moment a most difficult problem. It is so very easy to turn the hut tax now by growing cotton; the women and the children do the work, and the man, the lord of the household, looks on encouragingly, whilst occasionally lending a hand. The crop produced is sufficient to pay all necessary expenses for the year.[23]

However, the growing of cotton was initially regarded as an extension of women's traditional food-growing responsibilities, but it was not long before men took over cash crop production. The explanation for the shift was given by the Chief Agricultural Officer in 1910:

> Now a change is coming over the country ... The men have to do more, for women 'suffragettes' have appeared. They insist that, if they are not supplied with European clothing ... the banana supply for the family will stop; they will no longer cultivate, but go off and get work as labourers, and earn money with which to clothe themselves satisfactorily. In the face of this, a man wanting to live happily and with sufficient food has to supply the food and other luxuries demanded ... It is almost entirely owing to the fact that they are becoming Christians that the women ask for better treatment, and that the men have shown themselves willing to work as requested.[24]

Women were indeed refusing to cultivate the cotton, the cash proceeds of which belonged to their husbands. Cotton production was an added burden to their continued responsibility for subsistence production. This was in the more general context of men being freed from their obligations to women, and the erosion of women's rights to land within their natal kin group accompanying the privatization of land. Women's refusal to engage in cash crop production was more likely a sign of resistance to new forms of oppression and hardship created by changes in land tenure and familial relations, rather than a newly emerging 'suffragette consciousness' brought about by the Christianization process.

In 1909, the government added the system of 'kasanvu' – paid compulsory labour where each able-bodied male had to work one month at a rate determined by the government. Kasanvu was in addition to 'luwalo' – unpaid communal labour recruited by the chiefs. The despised kasanvu system remained in place until 1922, at which point the colonial office in London determined that the system in all its colonies was to be abolished. The end of kasanvu, coupled with the forced absorption of tens of thousands of Ugandans into the East African forces during Second World War, created acute labour shortages.[25] It was also during this time that Uganda was hit by epidemics of smallpox, dysentery, cerebro-spinal meningitis, and bubonic plague, followed after the war by influenza, further shrinking the supply of labour. Infectious diseases were directly attributable to the bad diet and living conditions experienced by migrant workers, but despite the serious labour shortages, employers relied on a high turnover rate to reduce the effects of illness on productivity. Doyal contends that this system made possible the maximum use of able-bodied migrants drawn from the peasant sector, while placing the burden of providing care for the sick back onto the same sector.[26]

Labour shortages led to the establishment of the Department of Labour in 1925, its functions being 'to recruit labour for the Government and to conduct it to the scene of employment; to study and improve the conditions under which labour was employed and the conditions under which the migrating labourer travelled along the supply routes'.[27] By 1925, more labour was coming from outside than inside the protectorate. According to Audrey Richards' study of migrant labour commissioned by the colonial government, the principal areas exporting unskilled labour within Uganda were the West Nile district and certain bordering localities in Kigezi; smaller numbers came from Ankole, Bugishu, Bunyoro, and Toro.[28] The majority of labourers, however, came from Ruanda-Urundi, reportedly to escape the Belgian system of compulsions that was considered far harsher than the British and, as well, during certain periods to escape famine. Large numbers also came from Tanganyika.[29] The study points to the consequences of the growing movement of migrants due to disease spread, 'the devastating and increasing disease which threatens every caravan and trade route', as the 1927 Annual Report of the Medical Department states.[30] The medical risks associated with the migrant labour system were well documented; deaths from dysentery, relapsing fever, spirillum fever, ulcers, malaria, and starvation were common.[31] Meagre measures were taken to improve the situation, such as the establishment of camps with food rations along the main routes.

Shortly after the establishment of the Department of Labour, the administration pressured the Buganda Lukiko to pass the Busulu and Nvujjo Act of 1927, an act which guaranteed male peasants the permanent use of their land, and greatly reduced the tribute paid to the land-owning chiefs. Tribute owed to the chiefs was now determined by the colonial government. The law also stipulated that when a peasant holder left a holding derelict for more than six months with neither wife nor other occupant, the mailo owner shall have the right to give the holding to another, and no compensation shall be payable. A wife had the right to live on a holding on the same terms as her husband, so long as he was alive and had not surrendered his interest in the holding. But the rights of a wife would lapse on the death of her husband, in which case the rights would pass on to the legal or customary heir, and all the crops would revert to the landowner.[32] The act encouraged peasant producers to increase their production of cotton and, later, coffee, giving them opportunities of enrichment at the expense of peasants in other areas of the protectorate. Colonial policy on labour recruitment assisted the Baganda by encouraging labour movement from other regions for work on Bugandan peasant coffee and cotton farms, and also by decreeing that labour could not be actively recruited from the Baganda region. Bugandan peasant farmers became important employers of African labour.[33] Labour was overwhelmingly male, short term, and seasonal, and peaked during the coffee and cotton harvests. In the plantation sector, the recruitment of migrant labour was based on the establishment of a nucleus of immigrants who worked from 6 months to 2 years at a time and then returned home for several months. The proportion of women to men coming from Rwanda was 1:5; from Tanganyika 1:11.9.[34]

Labour could be paid substantially under its value, given that the peasant sector remained the site of reproduction of the entire African labour force. As in neighbouring colonies, the viability of the migrant labour system depended upon its continued reproduction by the peasant sector, and it was largely women who provided the subsidizing function for male labour. Says Powesland of the colonial government's Report of the Committee of Enquiry into the Labour Situation in the Uganda Protectorate, 1938: 'The Government was not prepared to encourage – even cautiously – the formation of a class of workers exclusively dependent on wages, on account of the heavy wage and social service costs entailed, although it was willing to guide it, and to control it as far as possible in order that bad working or living conditions may not be avoidably created.'[35] The formation of a working class would serve to undermine capital accumulation, and urbanization would pose a challenge to indirect rule. The government would, however, deal with the 'evils' associated with the migrant labour system, by closing borders when epidemic disease threatened the labour supply, when famine conditions in other colonies threatened to provoke too great an influx of migrants, and by supervising immigrant routes and providing rations, fuel, and firewood at selected camps. When in 1928 and 1943 famine conditions in Ruanda-Urundi threatened to send many thousands of Ruandans over the border, the frontier was closed, the reason given that Uganda's famine reserves could be exhausted by the influx of those seeking work and food.[36]

Post-war economic development in Uganda was largely based on the Worthington Plan published in 1947 that called for an increase in productivity over the next 10 years 'at a rate much higher than population'.[37] According to Ahluwalia, labour policy did not change significantly, although the colonial government shifted to a policy that aimed at achieving labour stabilization as part of the new emphasis on industrialization.[38] An immigrant minority from India controlled the processing of export agriculture, marketing, and the evolving import-substituting industries. The development of secondary industries – textile, chemical, cement, and metal industries based on cheap power supplies – was made possible by the 1948 Owen Falls Hydroelectric Scheme in Jinja. Efforts, however, to stabilize labour remained futile, as a large number of immigrants continued to enter Uganda in search of short-term employment.[39] By 1950, the three main immigrant routes into Buganda were the Southwest route from Tanganyika and Ruanda-Urundi; the Eastern Route which carried immigrants from the Eastern Province of Uganda and the Kavirondo District of Kenya; and the Northern Route from the West Nile and the Sudan.[40] Peasant agriculture was to remain the backbone of the Ugandan economy until 1972.

Colonial social policy, health and gender

Certain 'problems' were created by the migrant labour system and by the deep disruption in systems of governance and production. Two main and interrelated concerns of the protectorate government brought about by economic and migratory transformation were the control of disease and the control of women. Health policy became a mechanism to shape the morality of the African population and to ensure its continued reproduction. Christian missionaries were the central figures in this regard. The policy largely failed. What it did succeed in doing, however, was introducing a moral framework that to this day competes alongside the residues of 'traditional' customary practices informing sexual behaviour.

A devastating epidemic of sleeping sickness between 1900 and 1920 left behind 'not only a group of doctors and scientists familiar with conditions in Uganda but also a pattern for administrative intervention in the health and lives of the protectorate's people by a system of local administration that oversaw public health, and a pattern of visiting medical commissions that advocated advanced and coercive therapies and population management'.[41] Carol Summers describes the gradual evolution of a public health policy that integrated both biomedical and ideological initiatives to reconstruct the African population. It was in part through public health policy that the administration sought to maintain indirect rule, avoid labour shortages, and prevent dissension or rebellion by the African population. Summers describes the social programmes of the protectorate as more than mere sideshows to the politics and economics of imperialism, but as integral to the holding of power.[42] One of the dominant issues debated by colonial authorities early in the history of the protectorate was the effects of the introduction of Christian values on tribal society. On the one hand, Christianity was seen to liberate women from the harshest aspects of 'traditional' patriarchal oppression. But on the other hand, it was also seen as contributing to the social and moral disintegration of Africans. Colonel Lambkin, an officer of the Royal Army Medical Corps, argued back in 1908 that the introduction of Christianity created moral problems stemming from the erosion of 'traditional' patriarchal authority, unleashing an uncontrolled female sexuality, an idea that became widespread throughout colonial East and Central Africa.[43] States Lambkin:

> The freedom enjoyed by women in civilized countries has gradually been won by them as one of the results of centuries of civilization, during which they have been educated... Women whose female ancestors had been kept under surveillance were not fit to be treated in a similar manner. They were, in effect, merely female animals with strong passions, to whom unrestricted opportunities for gratifying these passions were suddenly afforded.[44]

At least under traditional rule, women's dangerous passions had been kept in check! The unleashing of their 'dangerous passions' was seen to be fuelling the spread of venereal disease, high rates of which were reported throughout the protectorate through the entire colonial period. F. R. Bettley, in a report on gonorrhoea, syphilis, and chancroid in soldiers from East Africa, argued that Christianity and 'western civilization' had weakened traditional tribal control and the result was that prostitutes were wandering widely, plying their trade.[45] According to colonial health records, the rate of infection of syphilis among the Bugandan population was, in the early 1900s, 80 per cent[46] although the confusion of endemic yaws and gonorrhoea with syphilis probably exaggerated this statistic. Still, the British had recorded more deaths than births in the protectorate up until 1924. Cook observed that in Mengo Hospital between 1897 and 1907 rates of syphilis increased rapidly, with 80 per cent of patients in 1921 having at one time suffered from the disease.[47] Later in 1933, he reported that two out of three Baganda mothers had suffered from syphilis and that the percentage of abortions or premature births in women with active signs of the disease was in the range of 65 per cent.[48] In 1945, it was reported that STDs were having a significant negative impact on the birth rate, and were resulting in high levels of sterility among women. The census of 1948 showed that 24.4 per cent of Baganda women over the age of 45 had never had a child.[49]

Civil war, smallpox, cholera, sleeping sickness, and bubonic plague also contributed to keeping the recorded death rate above the birth rate.[50] However, population decline was mainly attributed to the extremely high prevalence of STDs that were considered a threat to the viability of the protectorate.[51] The chiefly elite of Buganda embraced the idea that what the country was experiencing was an epidemic of STDs caused by the promiscuity of uncontrolled women.[52] But the colonial administration viewed male sexuality as a more immediate problem because males appeared more autonomous in the conduct of their sexual relations given that men, rather than women, lived in the towns and constituted the wage labour force. Some colonial officials pointed to the system of labour migration as contributing to moral decay. In the absence of their husbands, women were perceived as committing adultery, fuelling the spread of STDs and procuring abortions that would lead to infertility. The issue was deflected back on women through an emerging public discourse on mother and child welfare and the construction of the ideal African family.[53] The administration tried to address the problems created by the migrant labour system through a medical and ideological campaign targeted at rural women. Through the cultivation of sexually monogamous, domesticated families and education in sexual self-control, the problem of the moral anarchy pervading Bugandan society would be resolved. Says Summers, 'officials and missionaries became increasingly intrusive as they examined bodies for lesions, condemned the moral state of sufferers and demanded repentance and then combined bodily care and reproductive evangelism in the maternity program'.[54] Mission-trained African midwives were central to this strategy, which attempted to redirect female sexuality to more wholesome directions, stressing the sanctity of family life and the mothering role. Young women were trained, and then sent out to villages not only to provide prenatal and birthing services, but also to preach monogamy and devotion to one's husband and children. And through their chaste behaviour, midwives were to set an example for the wider community.

But as Summers suggests, the tiny excess of births over deaths was not necessarily the result of STD treatment or midwives' care. Despite the rapid expansion of midwife training, only about 2000 of 16,000 live births registered in Buganda were attended by certified midwives.[55] Furthermore, many of the young midwives, who received a paltry income at best and little support, came to reject the basic tenets of their training, often exhibiting 'unchaste' behaviour. The policy was bound to fail given the context in which it was implemented. The social and moral frames within which Ugandans conceptualized sexual relations did not include the understanding of 'chastity' that the missionaries had in mind. But more importantly, the evolving patterns of single-gender labour migration and the increasing number of residentially separate spouses militated against the creation of chaste, monogamous nuclear families. The two most comprehensive reports on urbanization in Uganda during the colonial period are A. W. Southall and P. C. W. Gutkind's *Townsmen in the Making: Kampala and its Suburbs* published in 1957 and Walter Elkan's *Migrants and Proletarians: Urban Labour in the Economic Development of Uganda* published in 1960. Their rich descriptions of the evolution of urban life strongly support the argument that gender and familial relations were undergoing changes quite different from the ones that the missionaries had hoped for.

Apart from the European colonialists and the Asian merchant class, single African men peopled the towns. When women did move to the urban areas to escape the increasing difficulties or rural life, according to Southall and Gutkind, more often than not they came alone; it was rare that a man and a woman would come together. They describe the demographics of Kisenyi, the densest area of African labour settlement in Kampala, as 40 per cent women to 60 per cent men, this showed a higher proportion of women than was to be found anywhere else in the city.[56] There were also very few children, compared to the rural areas. The African population was highly mobile, indicated by the fact that only 20 per cent of the population had paid taxes in 2 years running. For the men, opportunities in the newly emerging industrial sector and in trades lured them into the towns, and some women came in turn to offer domestic and sexual services to these men, in the hopes of saving enough cash to establish themselves as independent businesswomen. A range of economic/sexual relationships evolved; for women, allowing them more autonomy than they would have in the countryside under the control of appointed chiefs; for men, offering them domestic services, companionship, and sex in the absence of their wives.

A similar situation is echoed in Elkan's descriptions of Jinja and Kampala as heterogeneous, its industrial labour forces being made up of short-term migrants. Two-thirds of the employees of Kampala and Jinja were considered foreigners, many from outside Uganda.[57] Levels of unskilled wages in the industries of Kampala and Jinja fell far below the minimum necessary to support a family for any length of time even under the direst poverty. Farm income, whether for subsistence or surplus, is 'a part of the family income no less than wages earned in employment'.[58] Men would stay in the cities, periodically returning to the villages to stock up on food rations and visit their families. States Elkan, 'leaving a family at home or on the farm is, in Africa, not incompatible with conjugal life in town and many of the ties which those who can afford it form with women in the town have about them a semblance of stability'.[59]

But, as previously stated, not all women remained in the countryside. The influx of women from the rural areas into the towns reflected the limits of rural chiefly control. With the absence of native courts in the cities, customary marriages and 'traditional family life' were not 'safeguarded' or provided for by law at all, as they were by the collaboration of chiefs and colonial authorities in the rural areas. Women and girls came to Kampala to escape intolerable conditions in the rural areas, or when their marriages ended and they were left destitute.[60] Hence the continuation of 'African promiscuity' and the high rates of STDs that continued relatively unabated into the independence period.

The social upheaval resulting from the introduction of the cash economy, the migrant labour system, and the erosion of the precolonial social/moral order could hardly be reversed through the moralizing projects of the missionaries. Independence brought further disruption to Ugandan society, but the system of governance characterized by Buganda sub-imperialism and competing systems of civil and traditional law underlies the tragedy of the immediate post-colonial period. If the colonial period established patterns of control and exploitation through labour, economic, and social policies, the immediate post-colonial period launched violent struggles to throw off the yoke of Baganda's 'sub-imperialism' and unleashed new inter-societal tensions. The post-colonial political arrangement was negotiated in haste and was not accepted by any of the major power blocs; Baganda nationalists declared it a sell-out and launched a violent rebellion which was suppressed by the army. One of the key young officers helping to put down the rebellion was none other than Idi Amin. The social forces underlying the epidemiology of HIV in Uganda can be seen, at least in part, as the outcome of Uganda's historical legacy.

The colonial legacy – vestiges of the bifurcated state, an economy and social system, functioning in part around single-gender labour migration, of women's tenuous legal and economic status – shaped the social context of HIV spread. Colonialism severed the links between community moral values and sexual behaviour, while at the same time shaping 'custom' and 'tradition' to serve its own ends. A system evolved where the urban areas represented freedom from the harshest aspects of chiefly rural control, while in the rural areas, custom was enforced by the native authorities and backed by the central state. The range of sexual and familial relationships that evolved can be viewed as a response to the disruptions of the colonial episode. History challenges the commonly held assumption of African sexuality as innately indiscriminate and free, and as part of the static realm of 'cultural behaviour' divorced from broader social and economic developments.

Uganda's independence

Most official accounts of Uganda at independence are very positive. Take, for example, the following description from the executive summary of the WB report, *Uganda: Growing Out of Poverty*:

> At independence (1962) Uganda had one of the most vigorous and promising economies in Sub-Saharan Africa, and the years following independence amply demonstrated this economic potential. Favoured with a good climate and fertile soil, the country was self-sufficient in food, with the agricultural sector being a large earner of foreign exchange. The manufacturing sector supplied the economy with basic inputs and consumer goods and was also a source of foreign exchange earnings through the export of textiles and copper. Export earnings not only financed the country's import requirements but also resulted in a current account surplus. Fiscal and monetary management was sound and the domestic savings rate averaged about 15 percent of GDP, enough to finance a respectable level of investment. Uganda's system of transportation was widely regarded as one of the best in SSA and included an effective network of railways, port and air transport. Uganda's social indicators were comparable to, if not better than, most countries in Africa. The country's health service had developed into one of Africa's best and pioneered many low cost health and nutrition programs. There existed a highly organized network of vaccination centres and immunization programs reached as much as 70 percent of the population. Although school enrolment was still low, Uganda's education system had developed a reputation for very high quality.[61]

It is difficult to dispute the facts contained in this description. Their effect is to create a snapshot of Uganda at independence as a viable society according to standard western measures – sound economic growth and levels of investment, good social indicators and infra-structural development. What is not mentioned is that household food security was tenuous at best – dependent on the exploitation of women's unpaid labour and strained by increasing competition between cash croppers and subsistence producers, and areas of the north frequently experienced famine. 'Africa's best' health care system was largely hospital-based and western-oriented, and the vast majority of people did not have access to the most basic constituents of health such as proper sanitation and clean water. And many diseases were endemic, such as malaria, hookworm, syphilis, yaws, TB, and gonorrhoea. The Ugandan diet was high in carbohydrates and low in protein and calcium, substantially due to the diversion of subsistence-producing land to cash cropping and the early introduction of the protein-scarce, perennial green banana as a dietary staple.[62] Uganda's 'very high-quality' education system was based on the British curriculum with limited provision of technical, vocational, or agricultural training, in essence geared to provide clerks and cadres of lower civil servants for the colonial administration.[63]

The description also implies that colonialism was essentially beneficial, and that Uganda's poverty, which it is to 'grow out of' with WB assistance, is a result of the immediate post-colonial period. The most common explanation for Uganda's fall into chaos is the coming to power by Idi Amin, rather than the legacy of a century of colonial rule and the social and cultural disruption it caused. Certainly, both are important and interrelated. Amin's brutal leadership is better understood in light of the geopolitical nature of polity and the state inherited at independence. Many of the inherent problems of the post-colonial Uganda state were not apparent in 1962, but became obvious as the years following independence unfolded.

Khadiagala describes the first civilian regime of Milton Obote as a 'grand post-colonial experiment' – an attempt to manage Uganda's cultural pluralism by balancing central control with dispersed mechanisms of local control and participation. 'State collapse began with the unravelling of this constitutional experiment.'[64] The 1962 constitution had allowed a measure of decentralization – the dispersal of power among predominant ethnic groups. This compromised Obote's ability to consolidate power. His ultimate strategy was to encroach on the powers of federated states through proscription of kingdoms and the imposition of a one-party state in 1967. He did this by increasing the power of the military and by using it against his civilian opponents. Military power became indispensable to Obote's rule. The central state increasingly limited the power of local groups, especially the Baganda, who struggled to maintain their autonomy. Amin was in essence a product of this gradual disintegration of the state. As the head of an army increasingly central to state power, he became all the more powerful. Obote tried to undercut Amin's position by building a countervailing force against the regular army, but ultimately failed, the result being that in January 1971, Amin and his men overthrew the Obote government.

The African country with the reputation for having a better opportunity of making rapid progress than all its neighbours instead became a worst-case scenario on the continent, the next two decades becoming further engulfed in multiple crises. Amin began with the brutal slaughter of large numbers of Acholi and Lango, and senior officers who failed to switch allegiances quickly enough. Between 1971 and 1986, it is estimated that approximately 800,000 people were murdered; 500,000 and 300,000 under the rule of Amin and Obote II respectively.[65] The 1970s saw a sharp decline in the health of Ugandans, brought about by the deterioration of the health and social infrastructure, and the fleeing of medical and health professionals from the country. Services decayed badly or ceased to exist. Vandalism and looting occurred in many hospitals and clinics, and the entire health administrative structure crumbled. The water and sanitary system crumbled, resulting in increases in water- and faecal-borne diseases.[66]

State collapse inevitably led to economic stagnation and rampant inflation. Between 1972 and 1980, Uganda's total GDP per capita continuously dropped, despite significant increases in international prices for Uganda's primary products. Amin's 'Economic War' resulted in the expulsion of the Asian community, as over 8700 properties were nationalized or transferred to the newly created 'Departed Asians Properties Custodial Board', including most of Uganda's manufacturing plants. Done in the name of 'Africanization', the move was disastrous for the economy as most of the professionals running the private sector were Asians. The Custodial Board allocated properties to Ugandans, but did little to ensure that they were maintained or that factories continued production. The Board instead became one of the mechanisms for institutionalized nepotism over the next two decades, with tenants changing with every regime.

The civil service began to take on an increasingly 'ethnic' character as government positions were granted to Amin's ethnic group from the northwest of the country. Unqualified relations and close associates of Amin were given positions of power within the civil service; leading to the virtual collapse of administrative capacity and the siphoning of budgets, and resulting in the disintegration of the health and education systems, and the general decay of basic infrastructure. The reality of daily life for the majority was household survival through any means. Violence became endemic, part and parcel of the evolving 'magendo economy', the informal economy based upon two reinforcing systems of economic controls: price controls on the sale of produce and an artificially high exchange rate. Producers of agricultural commodities received extremely low returns from their crops, while importers, with access to foreign exchange, imported commodities through formal channels to sell in the parallel market at many times their official value. The magendo economy was based on the smuggling of coffee, paraffin, sugar, and gold out of the country, vehicle spares and other necessities into the country and food within the country.[67] One's personal success depended upon connections with the military establishment and access to foreign exchange. A 'motley group of wheeler-dealers'[68] called the mafutamingi became central to the economy; a 'rapacious state-created, state protected stratum of big proprietors'.[69] Green describes the magendo economy as a 'brutally exploitative system which degrades, corrupts, deprives, and routinely kills'.[70]

The freezing of agricultural prices and the drawing of large quantities of cash crops into the black market had a particular importance in Buganda which supplied much of the food needs of the major towns of Kampala and Jinja,[71] as did Amin's Land Reform Decree in 1975, which repealed the 1928 Busulu and Enjujjo Law, removing security of tenure from (male) peasant producers. There was a shift away from support for peasant agriculture to the combination of landlords and wealthy bureaucrats. Peasants were now 'tenants-at-will' who could be evicted in the name of 'development'.[72] When Amin was finally ousted by a joint military force composed of Ugandan exiles and the Tanzanian army in 1979, the economy and the polity were shattered. Inflation was out of control and parastatals, which had been responsible for the marketing of cotton, coffee, and tea, had lost all credibility with the Ugandan peasantry. Milton Obote was reinstalled as the President in 1980 after what were perceived as fraudulent elections. In response to the rigging of these elections, Yoweri Museveni, a leader of one of the rebellious exile groups, went back to the bush and started a guerrilla war against Obote.

During his second term in office (1980–1985) known as the Obote II period, Obote had become even more dependent upon the army for support, and within a few years his power began to erode. Violence and human rights violations increased, inflation was rampant, and official exports continued to show increasing reliance on agricultural produce with an overall downward trend. Between 1973 and 1980, inflation was running at 45 per cent per annum; between 1980 and 1987, this rose to 95 per cent. Obote initially tried to solve his economic problems by printing more money, a strategy that resulted in even greater inflation.[73] Under the tutelage of the IMF and the WB, Obote embarked on a structural adjustment programme in 1981 but was unable to sustain any political commitment to the programme and was forced to abandon it within 3 years.[74] In 1985, he was ousted a second time by a military force, this time led by General Tito Okello. In the meantime, a protracted guerrilla war led by Museveni and his National Resistance Movement (NRM) was gaining in popular support. Okello tried to prevent Museveni coming to power by embarking on negotiations with him in Nairobi in 1985. But the insurgency continued to grow, and Museveni was joined by a number of other rebel forces.

The economic collapse continued unabated through this period. The neglect of agricultural production and the retreat of the state from rural areas in some instances strengthened peasant autonomy. In some places, informal household-food strategies such as the planting of cassava ensured survival, the exceptions being where the population was severely disturbed or displaced, such as the Luwero Triangle, West Nile, and Karamoja. In other areas, the breakdown in central authority augmented the free reign of local chiefs, fostering a climate for the economic coercion of the peasantry. An increased disdain for the central government, building on the general antipathy towards government fostered through colonialism, was one of the political and psychological legacies of the first two decades of independence.

It was also likely during this period that high levels of sexual violence targeted at women accompanied state brutality. Statistics on the extent of sexual violence against women are hard to come by for specific periods, but connections have been made between civil strife, war, and the systematic rape of women. A recent report by Human Rights

Watch titled 'Just Die Quietly: Domestic Violence and Women's Vulnerability to HIV in Uganda' reveals the extent of gender-based violence and the persistence of spousal rape, 'the result of historically persistent unequal power relations and restraints on women's equality and sexual autonomy'.[75] Spousal abuse is a reflection of prevailing economic, political, and social conditions.[76] Epstein states that 40 per cent of Ugandan women have been victims of sexual violence, including rape and coercion by husbands, boyfriends, as well as strangers.[77]

Okello was ousted from power by the National Resistance Army (NRA) in January 1986, 15 years to the day when Idi Amin had taken control. The shattered country that Museveni inherited was an ideal environment for the spread of HIV. The social upheaval created by two decades of violence and terror, the virtual absence of a social safety net throughout the country, pronounced gender inequality and sexual violence against women, and continuous population movement fuelled by violence and insecurity provided an ideal environment for the spread of HIV infection. The first wave of HIV spread occurred during this period of extreme instability.

Uganda's reconstruction

When Museveni and the NRM came to power, they did so 'in a climate of diminished popular faith in the capacity of the state to provide security... The dominant trend was institutional immobilism, creating uncertainty, loss of commitment to the common good, devaluation of human life, and mistrust of authority.'[78] The new regime adopted a ten-point programme emphasizing democracy, security, national unity, and the reconstruction of the economy. Museveni co-opted leading members of the old political parties into his broad-based government by giving them ministerial positions, a strategy aimed at allowing him to concentrate on rebuilding a disciplined national army and a functioning civil service. Political parties agreed to suspend partisan activities until the adoption of a new constitution, and in 1989 he established a commission for this purpose.[79]

Resistance Councils (RCs) were established throughout the country (today called LCs or Local Councils), evolving from the security structures that were put in place during the guerrilla war to maintain liberated territory. Mamdani explains that in order to gain the support of the peasantry against the Obote II regime, this form of power had to highlight the question about the rights of the peasantry in the institutions it created. Its starting point was the replacement of chiefship with the system of RCs and committees, with legislative and judicial powers.[80]

> The introduction of the Resistance Council and Committee system to the entire country in the post-1986 period was the single most important political achievement of the NRA/M, for this measure dismantled the indirect rule regime at the local level and replaced it with village self-governance. The chief was stripped of judicial, executive and legislative powers and reduced to the position of an administrative official.[81]

The 'Resistance Councils and Committees Statutes 1987' stated that a 'Resistance Council shall be a policy-making organ in its area of jurisdiction, and in particular shall, (a) identify local problems and find solutions thereto; (b) formulate and review development plans; (c) at the district level, pass annual estimates; (d) make bye-laws in accordance with section 25 of the Statute; and (e) perform such other functions as may be delegated to it by the minister'.[82] The RCs were conceived as the vehicles for grassroots participation in Museveni's 'no-party democracy', a system for amalgamating all forces irrespective of past political affiliation. In the pyramidal resistance committee structure, elections were held at the lowest levels to elect members of the village-level RC; from there, the four other levels would be appointed from the ground up.

The empowerment of local communities through the RC structures has had a mixed record. In the early 1990s, in some of the areas surrounding Kampala and Jinja, people expressed a common sentiment that although they did not want to dispense with the RC structures all together, they resented having to participate when they perceived that certain local, strong men dominate, or that in the context of generalized poverty, participation brought little reward. 'People attended the meetings at the beginning, when they were given sugar' was the statement of the RC 1 chair in a peri-urban community. In some areas, the local-level RCs have become another means of accumulation for those in control. The following sentiments of a young woman in Jinja were shared by the people listening to our conversation:

> The time is coming when we will fear to talk to the RCs – they are no longer our people. We are forced to pay UgShs 200 a month for security. If we havn't paid they will knock on your door at midnight and demand the money. In my home village, you have to have a resident card that costs UgShs 400 and some boys were beaten because they didn't have one. The RCs can charge whatever they want.[83]

There is also anecdotal evidence that the RC system has been used against women to the extent that 'traditional' means of dealing with domestic abuse and sexual violence has meant in some instances that men's crimes have gone unpunished.

Local RCs, not simply as structures for grassroots democracy, have also become the means to mobilize 'voluntary' labour and to provide basic social services. At the central level, the basic contradictions of the post-colonial state have combined with the antistatism and neoliberal economic model of the IMF and the WB. The contradictions have reached far out to the countryside, where peasant communities have been drawn into the system in a way that has promoted and facilitated the expansion of privatization and the deepening of capitalism. Uganda's structural adjustment programme designed by the WB and the IMF has borne all the standard features of SAPs across the continent: deregulation of economic and commercial activities; massive public sector cutbacks; trade liberalization; the revision of investment codes and profit repatriation; the renegotiation of debt arrears; and a commitment to let the currency float on the international market.[84]

Conditions in Uganda since independence were extremely favourable for the spread of STD – population movement, war, marital instability and gender competition, and little in the way of a social safety net. Rural–urban linkages, formed during the colonial period, deepened further as many wage earners resorted to growing their own food or collecting it from rural-based relatives. Museveni's coming to power corresponded to the recognition of HIV as a serious health problem, but the epidemic had taken hold prior to 1986. The shattered polity inherited by the new regime was unprepared for the magnitude of the epidemic, but it can be said that it responded in a way unmatched on the African continent.

The HIV epidemic

In the early 1990s, the distribution of HIV in Africa stretched west across the continent along the equator, with the highest rates found closest to Lake Victoria both in rural and in urban areas. To the north and south, prevalence figures were lower except in urban and peri-urban areas situated close to major transportation routes in Kenya, Tanzania, Zambia, and Malawi, although infection rates were also on the rise in certain urban areas in southern and West Africa. To the west of Lake Victoria, the belt of high prevalence included the nations of equatorial Central Africa, especially Rwanda, Congo, and Burundi.

Anecdotal and observational evidence places the introduction of HIV to Uganda around the mid-1970s, corresponding to the contemporary period of turmoil. A small number of people living close to the shores of Lake Victoria in the district of Rakai were stricken with a disease that caused gradual wasting and was unresponsive to treatment. The first deaths are said to have occurred around 1981 in Goma, also known as Kasensero, a small fishing village on the shore of the lake, the date corresponding roughly to the beginning of Obote's second rule. This was about the same time that the new disease was first detected in North America. Little was known about the disease. HIV remained undetected for some time, given the political instability and the virtual absence of health services. The first deaths were likely attributed to other endemic diseases common to the region or to supernatural causes.

'Slim', as the disease was commonly called, was concentrated in certain areas. People in the trading centres of Rakai, Masaka, and Mpigi Districts in particular, and in Kampala and Jinja seemed to be falling sick from the mysterious disease that led to wasting and death from pneumonia-like symptoms. It was not until 1987 that it was proposed that a system be put in place to assess serosurveys and surveillance data. Serosurveys that had been carried out in 1986 indicated the following levels among test groups: long-distance truckers, 33 per cent; barmaids in North Rakai, 86 per cent; TB patients in

Kampala, 30 per cent; and women at prenatal clinics, 13.5 per cent.[85] The initial data pointed to the concentration of infection in particular areas and cohorts. Long-distance truckers, barmaids, and prostitutes exhibited the highest levels, but deaths of soldiers in the military were causing concern, with estimates that 40 per cent of soldiers carried the virus.[86] The level of infection in Rakai caused grave alarm, and was reported internationally, placing Uganda on the map as the global AIDS epicentre. Twenty sentinel survey sights were established by 1989. The sights were geographically distributed throughout the country, and the data was to be derived from antenatal clinic attendees. It was given that the data would not necessarily reflect the magnitude of infection, given that a high proportion of the population never attended health clinics. The general accuracy and completeness of reporting was also questionable, and HIV/AIDS was being diagnosed clinically, the cost of blood testing out of reach of the ACP.

But in addition to the surveillance activities of the ACP, other research projects were established throughout the country to monitor the progression of the epidemic. The Rakai Project, a sero-epidemiology project to study the dynamics of HIV and the effect of health education, was established in the worst-hit district of Rakai.[87] The Medical Research Council (MRC/UK) through the ODA provided institutional support to the UVRI to carry out a range of projects on HIV transmission and risk factors such as social and behavioural studies related to HIV/AIDS interventions. US-based World Learning Inc. established a number of projects that included HIV testing. The data, therefore, comes from a variety of disparate sources.

What the data indicated was a geographic pattern of infection that corresponded to the movement of migrant labourers, and reflected unequal gender relations. Untreated STDs – a more general symptom of the absence of basic health care and the widespread practice of self-diagnosis and prescribing – fuelled the spread of HIV. One's likelihood of becoming HIV infected increases as much as eight times in the presence of an untreated STD. The concentration of infection in the crescent around Lake Victoria and in areas of intense instability pointed to the relationship between HIV spread and historical and contemporary social transformations in the region. The location of the first known infections was the beginning of an important trade route that begins in the Rakai District and runs through the districts of Masaka and Mpigi, where Kampala is situated. This is one of the three routes that Audrey Richards documented in her study of migrant labour commissioned by the colonial government. During the colonial period, labourers and traders from Rwanda and Tanganyika followed this southwest route. During the immediate post-independence period, significant movement also continued along the Eastern Route from Kenya into Jinja and on to Kampala. Population movement along the third major migration route, originating in the north from the West Nile into the Sudan, was cut off during the Amin and Obote years – the war in this instance slowing down the flow of migrant labourers from the north into Kampala. High rates have also been found in areas of more intense destabilization such as Luwero and Gulu. Luwero bore the brunt of Obote's second rule; estimates of the casualties of war in the area known as the Luwero Triangle between 1981 and 1985 range from 100,000 to 1/2 million,[88] and to this day Gulu remains an area characterized by the extreme brutality of rebel movements and an active slave trade in children originating in the Sudan. Throughout the Amin and Obote years, people escaped alternately to the villages when the towns became too dangerous and to rural centres and urban areas when the villages were deemed unsafe. In 1979, the combination of an invading army moving through the area from the Tanzanian border together with fatalities amongst local men meant that there were additional opportunities for the disease to spread. The association of rebel activity and banditry with the rape and sexual abuse of women was commonly reported during Amin's and Obote's rule, and violence against women and girls was intense in the war-torn areas. Relations of oppression were fostered by a political climate that eroded collective and cooperative values, giving way to an ethic of individual survival by any means. Prevalence was lowest in the farming areas where the population has been relatively more settled and there had been few disturbances, such as Moyo and Kotido.

General seroprevalence data mask the microvariations in geographic incidence. A cohort study of the Rakai District was carried out between 1990 and 1991, the results of which were published in 1994. The district had a population of 385,000 living in three geographic strata – the main-road trading centres of Kyotera, Kalisizo, and Lyantonde (5 per cent) which serve local, domestic, and international traffic; intermediate trading villages on secondary roads (4 per cent) which act as foci for local communications; and rural agricultural villages (91 per cent) off main and secondary roads. The data showed that HIV prevalence in the trading centres was 35 per cent; in the intermediate trading villages, 23.1 per cent; and in the rural villages, 13.0 per cent.[89] HIV-related deaths occurred disproportionately in trading-centre residents compared with residents of the intermediate and rural villages. The age and sex structure of the cohort population was consistent with the national census data for Rakai – significant in this regard was that there were approximately 25 per cent fewer male residents in the 15–20 age group compared with females in the same age group due to male out-migration. The adult trading-centre population had 27 per cent more young women aged 15–39 as a result of work opportunities provided by the bars, lodges, and shops.

The prevalence of HIV infection among the cohorts was lower in men than in women; 15 vs. 24 per cent. Moreover, deaths among HIV-infected adult women occurred at a younger age: 56 per cent of the female deaths occurred between 15 and 19 years of age compared with 37 per cent of deaths among HIV-infected adult men. The report indicates that higher rates of HIV infection are found among better-educated persons and those working in non-agricultural occupations; however, the data on income and formal education was not disaggregated by gender. Evidence suggests that this is the case for males, but not females. A study that was part of a larger ethnographic project in one of the three trading centres was carried out in 1992, focusing on women's occupations, income potentials, and personal sexual and HIV-related risks associated with their jobs. The most common low-income generating activities for women were cultivation, selling food, or working as barmaids. Most women lacked resources and had migrated to the community in search of employment and better life. A key finding of the study was that in a setting with many migratory men, there were considerable pressures on impoverished women to supplement their incomes by exchanging sex for money or other forms of support.

A major factor that most respondents associated with women's risky sexual behaviour was low pay. The prevalence of AIDS makes questions of economic survival more difficult for women in the community. At the same time, selling sex is one of the quickest and lowest capital expenditure strategies for income generation... In the public mind, most barmaids and restaurant waitresses are perceived as 'bamalaya' (prostitutes) because of their work-related combination of low pay and frequent contact with men.[90]

Spread of HIV was also attributed to the migration of widows from Rakai to other places after the death of their husbands. Most widows remain in their homes, supporting themselves and their children, but others, chased off their land by brothers of their husbands or unable to cope with rural poverty, sought access to land from a brother or father or sought to remarry or migrate to urban areas. Despite women's legal right to own land, in practice it remains the case that most women have only use rights to land obtained through their relation to a man or through consanguinity.[91] The attitude persists that a woman in her own right should not own land.

The social relations set in the local politics of survival in the initial area of epidemic focus, in particular Rakai and Masaka, were ideal for the efficient spread of the virus. What is considered 'rampant promiscuity' can be better understood in the light of the social and economic disruption caused by the Amin years, in this particular region reflected in the politics of the magendo economy. The gender dimensions of the crisis arise from the interplay of a number of historical factors discussed previously: women's tenuous legal position regarding property and inheritance; their marginalization in the formal economy; and the intransigence of an ideology of men's ownership of women's productive and reproductive labour. Men and women were differentially drawn into the magendo economy with consequences for HIV spread, illicit economic activity in the area having a serious destabilizing effect on the already unequal balance between men and women. Men who participated in the trade had grossly inflated incomes compared to women who remained subsistence producers, and within this were largely excluded from the economic security of owning land. Women's landlessness and insecurity of title meant that they did not have a share directly in the economic boom, particularly as the main cash crop, coffee, remained largely under male control. One of the few ways in which women could gain access to cash and goods appearing in the system was through sexual servicing.[92] Women gained access to economic resources through different types of sexual relationships with men, providing a range of domestic services including preparing food and brewing beer, providing lodging as well as sex and companionship.

The pattern of infection indicated a movement of the virus from the trading centres into the cities, and outward to the rural areas. In the latter case, HIV-infected men and women were returning back to their home villages for medical care, often spreading the virus. HIV was also spread by men returning to their home villages for periodic visits from areas of labour concentration such as Jinja and Kampala. In Kampala, home to approximately 25 per cent of the HIV-infected population, a common explanation was that urban life had led to the breakdown of moral codes governing sexual relations in the village. On closer examination the picture takes on slightly more complexity. Rather than the freedom of 'city life', the situation can be better explained in the historical nature of the relationship between the urban and the rural forged through colonialism, and the patterns of single gender migration and gender imbalance found in the urban areas. During the colonial period, urban areas became a place of economic opportunity and escape for some women who could no longer cope with the added economic burdens placed on them by the colonial economy and with the social control of despotic chiefs. But most Africans inhabiting the city were male. In the case of male migrants, the absence of wives was compounded by the fact that their new environment was almost exclusively masculine. The unequal sex ratio made it difficult for men to establish stable sexual relationships with women, and encouraged prostitution. More recent movements are continuities of patterns established during the colonial period, although population movement has been exacerbated by recent economic crises and by war and banditry.

For some women, the difficulties they continue to encounter in gaining employment and access to capital have established the various forms of sex selling. Opportunities are many, given the large numbers of single African men in the urban areas, and the phenomenon of having a 'free marriage' in town and a wife in the village. A socio-economic household survey of Jinja pointed to the continued fluid movement of people from city to countryside as a structural aspect of the low-wage economy and the very poor provision of social services. Of 400 households surveyed, 26 per cent had regular ties to 'the village', which included an economic relationship – food, leasing of land, another spouse, or grandparents taking care of children. A not-uncommon familial form was residentially separate spouses or partners who move according to economic opportunities, but have a base in the village – in this way, members of a household, who as individuals are marginalized, can pool resources and spread costs.

In the case of migrating husbands away from home, 'free marriages' or fluid domestic/sexual arrangements in the cities are common. Little has changed, to the extent that the subsistence sector still continues to subsidize cash crop production for export and wages in the industrial and public sectors. The extreme difficulty of living on a wage in Uganda means that men and women engage in a variety of economic activities. Urban dwellers depend on the produce from their villages to augment food that is purchased using their wages. Female-headed households – in Jinja the figure approached 30 per cent in the mid-1990s – are particularly vulnerable. Over half the households had a monthly combined income of UgShs 30,000; approximately Can$30, from which they paid for food, rent, transport, water, charcoal, school fees, and medical expenses. In almost all these cases, monthly expenditures vastly exceeded income, but it was difficult to discern where the money was coming from. In these circumstances, even the cost of condoms was prohibitive. These are the words of a 27-year-old government employee living in the low-income area of Walukuba: 'A smartly dressed woman came and asked us questions to find out if we would be willing to pay for condoms, of course, we are all willing to pay, just give us the money, and we will purchase the condoms.'

A study carried out in 1992 examined the socio-cultural factors that influence sexual risk behaviour among Baganda women in Kampala. In this case, the women are not an established 'risk group'. A sample of 130 women were recruited from a paediatric follow-up clinic, with a mean age of 21 years, and half HIV positive and half HIV negative. Their own perception of risk stemmed from their fear that men were generally unfaithful and it was socially acceptable for them to have many sexual partners. The vast majority of women claimed to be practicing monogamy or abstaining from sex altogether, but there was a general understanding that women do in fact have difficulty in this regard. The cases rather than the controls were more likely to state that women have outside sexual partners because of economic need: 72 vs. 54 per cent respectively. Another interesting finding was that of the cases, 21.5 per cent described their marital status as 'visiting unions' as opposed to 10 per cent of the controls, indicating that their men come and go. Ninety-Seven per cent of cases and ninety-five per cent of controls said that they were taking measures to protect themselves, but they also stated that they remain at risk of infection because they think that their partners are not faithful.[93]

The March 1996 Situational Summary of the HIV/AIDS Surveillance Report showed declining HIV trends in five urban sites; seroprevalence rates on average dropping from 16 per cent in 1993 to 14 per cent in 1995;[94] since then, there have been steady declines to present rates of, on average, 6.5 per cent. One of the chief epidemiologists with the ACP claimed that initial declines in HIV prevalence were likely due to the 'saturation effect' – the epidemic had peaked because people who had died of AIDS were more than those spreading HIV infection. Most people have witnessed the deaths of friends and family, a factor that is positively correlated with sustained change in sexual behaviour. However, HIV levels in some areas are now climbing; evidence suggesting that the decline in prevalence may be waning.[95]

It is indeed the case that the Ugandan response to HIV/AIDS was unmatched on the continent at the time. Uganda has become the model to emulate. The next chapter examines Uganda's multisectoral and broad-based strategy – its successes as well as its weaknesses. But I am also interested in the ways in which the 'success' of the strategy has been defined, and how Uganda's ACP has on the one hand failed to challenge persistent and systemic gender inequalities which continue to fuel the epidemic and render women responsible for 'mitigation', and on the other how it has fit into the broader neoliberal agenda embraced by the state.

Notes

1. Megan Vaughan, *Curing their Ills, Colonial Power and African Illness* (California: Stanford University Press, 1991) 144.
2. Jean-Francois Bayart, *The State in Africa: The Politics of the Belly* (London: Longman, 1993) 20.
3. Bayart, 20.
4. A. B. Mukwaya, *Land Tenure in Buganda: Present-Day Tendencies* (Kampala: Eagle Press, 1953) 15.
5. Thomas Taylor, 'The Establishment of a European Plantation Sector Within the Emerging Colonial Economy of Uganda, 1902–1919', *International Journal of African Historical Studies* 19.1 (1986): 39.
6. Phares Mutibwa, *Uganda Since Independence* (Kampala: Fountain Publishers, 1992) 5.

7. Mukwaya, 15.

8. Ibid., 15.

9. Ibid., 32.

10. Nakanyike Musisi, 'Women, Elite Polygyny and Buganda State Formation', *Signs* 16.4 (1991): 789.

11. Mahmood Mamdani, *Citizen and Subject: Contemporary Africa and the Legacy of Late Colonialism* (New Jersey: Princeton University Press, 1996) 52.

12. Mamdani, *Citizen*, 60.

13. Ibid., 50.

14. See, for example, Margaret Jean Hay and Marcia Wright, eds, *African Women and the Law: Historical Perspectives* (Boston: Boston University Papers on Africa, 1982) and Martin Chanock, 'Making Customary Law: Men, Women and Courts in Colonial Northern Rhodesia' in the same volume; also by Chanock, *Law, Custom and Social Order: The Colonial Experience in Malawi and Zambia* (Cambridge: Cambridge University Press, 1985).

15. Mamdani, *Citizen*, 122.

16. Ibid., 166.

17. Taylor, 37.

18. Ibid., 50.

19. D. P. S. Ahluwalia, *Plantations and the Politics of Sugar in Uganda* (Kampala: Fountain Publishers, 1995) 101.

20. See, for example, Claire Robertson and Iris Berger, eds, *Women and Class in Africa* (New York: Holmes and Meier, 1986); Achola Pala Okeyo, 'Daughters of the Lakes and Rivers: Colonization and the Land Rights of Luo Women', *Women and Colonization: Anthropological Perspectives*, eds M. Etienne and E. Leacock (New York: Praeger, 1980) 186–214; Mona Etienne, 'Women and Men, Cloth and Colonization: The Transformation of Production–Distribution Relations among the Baule' in the same volume, 214–38; Nancy J. Hafkin and Edna J. Bay, eds, *Women in Africa: Studies in Social and Economic Change* (Stanford: Stanford University, 1976).

21. Mamdani, *Citizen*, 120.

22. Ibid., 17.

23. Qtd in Audrey Richards, ed., *Economic Development and Tribal Change: A Study of Immigrant Labour in Buganda* (Cambridge: W. Heffer and Sons, 1952) 19.

24. Richards, *Economic*, 20–21.

25. Taylor, 55.

26. Doyal, 114–15.

27. P. G. Powesland, 'History of the Migration in Uganda', *Economic Development and Tribal Change: A Study of Immigrant Labour in Buganda*, ed. Audrey Richards (Cambridge: W. Heffer and Sons, 1952) 29.

28. Powesland, 43.

29. Audrey Richards, 'The Travel Routes and the Travellers', *Economic Development and Tribal Change: A Study of Immigrant Labour in Buganda*, ed. Audrey Richards (Cambridge: W. Heffer and Sons, 1952) 53.

30. Qtd in Powesland, 58.

31. Powesland, 58.
32. Mukwaya, 58.
33. Mutibwa, 7.
34. Richards 'Travel', 64.
35. Powesland, 45.
36. Ibid., 47.
37. Ibid., 48.
38. Ahluwalia, 141.
39. Ibid., 141.
40. Richards 'Travel', 53.
41. Carol Summers, 'Intimate Colonialism: The Imperial Production of Reproduction in Uganda, 1907–1925', *Signs* 16.4 (1991): 789.
42. Summers, 806.
43. Vaughan, 132.
44. Qtd in Vaughan, 133.
45. F. R. Bettley, 'Venereal Disease Control in East African Command', *Journal of the Royal Army Medical Corps* 85.3 (1945): 109–16.
46. Vaughan, 132.
47. Alexander Cooke, 'The Treatment of Ante-natal Syphilis', *East Africa Medical Journal* 6.1 (1929).
48. Alexander Cooke, 'The Influence of Obstetrical Conditions on Vital Statistics in Uganda', *East African Medical Journal* 9.11 (1933): 316–30.
49. F. Bennett, 'Venereal Diseases', *Uganda Atlas of Disease Distribution*, eds Hall and Langlands (1968), cited in Bernadette Olowo-Freers and Tom Barton, 'In Pursuit of Fulfillment: Studies of Cultural Diversity and Sexual Behavior in Uganda: An Overview Essay and Annotated Bibliography', unpublished report (Kampala, 1992) 52.
50. Summers, 787.
51. Ibid., 788.
52. Vaughan, 139.
53. Ibid., 130.
54. Summers, 806.
55. Ibid., 804.
56. A. W. Southall and P. C. Gutkind, *Townsmen in the Making: Kampala and its Suburbs* (Kampala: East African Institute of Social Research, 1957) 28.
57. Walter Elkan, *Migrants and Proletarians: Urban Labour in the Economic Development of Kampala* (London: Oxford University Press, 1960) 20.
58. Elkan, 135.
59. Ibid., 137.
60. Southall and Gutkind, 71.
61. World Bank, *Uganda: Growing Out of Poverty* (Washington D.C.: World Bank, 1993) xi.
62. C. O'Manique, 'Traditional Therapies and Biomedicine in Uganda', International Health Exchange Project Reports No. 3 (Ottawa: 1989) 71–84.
63. Oliver Furley, 'Education in Post-independence Uganda: Change amidst Strife', *Uganda Now: Between Decay and Development*, eds H. B. Hansen and M. Twaddle (London: James Currey, 1988) 176.

64. Gilbert M. Khadiagala, 'State Collapse and Reconstruction in Uganda', *Collapsed States: The Disintegration and Restoration of Legitimate Authority*, ed. William Zartman (London: Lynne Rienner, 1995) 35.
65. J. B. Mugaju, ed., *Uganda's Decade of Reforms 1986–1996* (Kampala: Fountain Publishers, 1996) 18–19.
66. D. Dunlop and S. Scheyer, 'Health Services and Development in Uganda', *Crisis in Uganda: The Breakdown of Health Services*, eds Paul Cole and Paul Wiebe (Oxford: Pergamon, 1985) 31.
67. Tony Barnett and Piers Blaikie, *AIDS in Africa: Its Present and Future Impact* (London: Belhaven Press, 1992) 72.
68. Vali Jamal, 'Inequalities and Adjustment in Uganda', *Development and Change* 22.2 (1991): 321.
69. Mahmood Mamdani, 'Uganda: Contradictions of the IMF Programme and Perspective', *Development and Change* 21 (1990): 434.
70. Reginald Green, 'Magendo in the Political Economy of Uganda: Pathology, Parallel System or Dominant Sub-mode of Production?' Discussion Paper 165, Institute of Development Studies (University of Sussex, 1981) 1.
71. Green, 1.
72. Mamdani 'Uganda', 453.
73. K. Sarwar Lateef, 'Structural Adjustment in Uganda: The Initial Experience', *Changing Uganda: The Dilemmas of Structural Adjustment and Revolutionary Change*, eds H. B. Hansen and M. Twaddle (London: James Currey, 1991) 21.
74. E. O. Ochieng, 'Economic Adjustment Programs in Uganda 1985–89', *Changing Uganda: The Dilemmas of Structural Adjustment and Revolutionary Change*, eds H. B. Hansen and M. Twaddle (London: James Currey, 1991) 44.
75. Human Rights Watch, 'Just Die Quietly: Domestic Violence and Women's Vulnerability to HIV', *Human Rights Watch Report* 15.15(a) (Aug. 2003): 9.
76. Human Rights Watch, 3.
77. Helen Epstein, 'AIDS: The Lesson of Uganda', *New York Review of Books* XLVIII.11 (5 July 2001): 20.
78. Khadiagala, 39.
79. Ibid., 39.
80. Mamdani, *Citizen*, 200–1.
81. Ibid., 215.
82. GOU, *The Resistance Councils and Committees Statute, 1987* (Entebbe: Government Printers, 1987) 79.
83. Excerpt from an interview in Jinja, 30-year-old female, Sept. 1992.
84. Christopher Gombay, 'Eating Cities: The Politics of Everyday Life in Kampala, Uganda', PhD thesis, University of Toronto, 1997, 123.
85. GOU/Ministry of Health, *ACP Proposals for a Five Year Action Plan 1987–1994* (Entebbe, Mar. 1987) 46.
86. Extracted from field notes of an interview with Dr Asiimwe-Okiror, epidemiologist, ACP (Aug. 1992).
87. This project was funded by USAID and the Rockefeller Foundation through the National Institutes of Allergy and Infectious Disease (US), and was implemented through Columbia University, the Uganda Ministry of Health and the Institute of Public Health, Makerere University.

88. Cole P. Dodge and Magne Raundalen, eds, *War, Violence and Children in Uganda* (Great Britain, 1987) 3.
89. Nelson Sewankambo *et al.*, 'Demographic Impact of HIV Infection in Rural Rakai District Uganda: Results of a Population-based Cohort Study', *AIDS* 8.12 (Dec. 1994): 1707–13.
90. Nakuti, J. *et al.*, 'If we Fear AIDS, What Will We Eat? Women's Struggle for Economic Independence in a Rural Uganda Lorry Stop', conference paper, 7th International Conference on AIDS in Africa (Yaounde, 8–11 Dec. 1992).
91. Barnett and Blaikie, 77.
92. Ibid., 77–78.
93. J. McGrath *et al.*, 'Anthropology and AIDS: The Cultural Context of Sexual Risk Behaviour Among Urban Women in Kampala, Uganda', *Social Science and Medicine* 36.4 (1993): 429–39.
94. Government of Uganda STD/AIDS Control Programme, Ministry of Health, *HIV/AIDS Surveillance Report March 1996* (Entebbe: Government Printers, 1996). The selected sights were Nsambya, Rubaga (both in Kampala), Mbarara, Jinja, Tororo, and Mbale.
95. Human Rights, 8.

5
The Uganda 'Success Story'

As the capital of one of Africa's 'fastest growing economies', Kampala appears booming and vibrant. Many of the roads are in good repair, old buildings have been painted and windows replaced, and new construction is evident. New stores, restaurants, boutiques, and nightclubs have been opened, and hotels, many renovated, are doing a steady business. A growing population of expatriates is visible, reflecting the stability that has allowed for the growth of international business and foreign development assistance. The stock exchange is located in a busy downtown office building. Other signs of progress are the European bakery, the home-made pasta shop, the mini-market that sells imported food from Europe – a big change compared to a decade and a half before, when Kampala was quiet, the buildings derelict, the streets pot-holed, and there was little evidence of commerce or an international presence. But on closer observation, Kampala still shows some signs of 'underdevelopment'. Sprawling neighbourhoods of small houses built of clay and corrugated iron continue to house many of Kampala's 'middle class'. The 2003 UN Development Report places 82.2 per cent of the Ugandan population below the income poverty line of $1 a day, and 48 per cent have no access to an improved water source.[1] Access to adequate health facilities is still out of reach for 50 per cent of the population. Life is certainly better for many people than it was in the days of Amin and Obote, but the wealth stemming from Uganda's 'successful' economic liberalization has not quite yet 'trickled down'. And zones of conflict remain in the north and southwest of the country, where much of the population continue to live in terror. In this light, AIDS is just one of a number of problems shaping the politics of daily life in Uganda, deepening for many of its citizens' already existing poverty and human insecurity.

The Uganda response to HIV/AIDS is widely touted as the African AIDS success story and the model to emulate. Surveillance data since 1993 has indicated a decline in HIV prevalence throughout the country, from an estimated peak of 29.4 per cent in 1992 (based on data from antenatal clinic attendees) to a level of 11.25 per cent in 2000.[2] This drop is attributed to the prevention efforts of the Ugandan government and the donor community. The reasons for Uganda's success in lowering prevalence rates, however, are not altogether clear, as evidence seemed to suggest only marginal changes in sexual behaviour by 1993. Data collected by the ACP and various donor projects did not point to sweeping and sustained changes in sexual behaviour. Also difficult to deem a success is Uganda's response in addressing the effects of HIV/AIDS-related morbidity and mortality on agricultural production, labour scarcity, and more generally on household survival and reproduction of the rural poor, despite a decade of calls for interventions to mitigate the deep impacts of HIV/AIDS. Despite a focus on the 'empowerment of women', mounting evidence points to marriage as the largest risk women today in Uganda of contracting HIV. According to an August 2003 Human Rights Watch Report, married women are most vulnerable to HIV infection because of domestic violence and unwanted sexual relations, and the pervasive acceptance throughout state institutions and society, in general, that married women are their husband's property. The report states that 'despite a rhetorical commitment to women's rights, the Ugandan government has ignored the role of violence, and, in particular, unwanted sexual relations in marriage, in exposing them to HIV infection'.[3] In a largely agricultural economy, where women do not own land but are responsible for 70 to 80 per cent of all agricultural work, the burden of care has fallen on the 'private sector' – overwhelmingly women in the 'private' household – resulting in intensive pressure on their labour time, as they simultaneously struggle to care for the sick and produce food for their families. Where women have also produced food for the market, their marketed food production has declined, leaving them without an independent source of cash income. And finally, life-saving ARV treatment in Uganda is out of the question for all but a tiny minority – the cost of one month's treatment roughly equal to annual per capita income. In this light, Uganda's success can be seen as, at best, partial.

The period from 1985 to 1990 saw the institutional consolidation of the ACP in Uganda and the proliferation of agencies in the AIDS sector; the emphasis of prevention and care on medical interventions and mass education campaigns to promote sexual behaviour change. The next phase in Uganda, beginning in the early 1990s, saw a growing emphasis on the 'multifaceted' nature of the epidemic which continues to this day, reflected in the emergence of the UAC in 1992 and Uganda's multisectoral strategy, its most recent articulation, The National Strategic Framework for AIDS Activities 2000/01–2005/06.

Circumscribing the response to HIV/AIDS is the broader macro-economic policy framework within which the response has evolved, and this is where my analysis begins. I then discuss the formation of the Uganda Ministry of Health (MOH) ACP, the structural problems confronted by its implementation, and the reasons behind the evolution of the 'multisectoral strategy'. Since the beginning of the ACP, we see a gradual shift to a more 'community-based' and 'multi-sectoral' programme, reflecting a growing concern over the social and economic consequences of the epidemic, as well as the decentralization programme of the government introduced in 1992 which in theory was to create increased decision-making and control of resources at the district level. At the same time, the multisectoral strategy has conformed to the broader social policy agenda of the GOU, shaped significantly by the IMF and the WB. My basic argument is that the boundaries of the policy response have been tightly circumscribed by the neo-liberal economic and social agenda; an agenda which valorises privatization and production for the market, while devaluing the activities and relations that fall outside the market. AIDS is not only a health crisis; it is also a crisis in the reproduction of the conditions of daily life.

The context: the national economy and health policy

The macroeconomic policy framework within which Uganda's multisectoral strategy has evolved was first articulated in 'The Way Forward Macroeconomic Strategy 1990–1995' formulated by the Ministry of Finance, Planning and Economic Development (Uganda) (MFPED). 'The Way Forward' was a macroeconomic framework designed to create 'an independent, integrated self-sustaining economy'.[4] It centred on export promotion to increase foreign exchange earnings, prudent budgeting, and disciplined expenditure. The framework attributed Uganda's economic problems to domestic policy weaknesses, in particular, a shortage of savings in the banking system because of negative real interest rates due to inflation that in turn was related to the excessive printing of money to finance budget deficits. This – along with an inefficient and complicated system of taxation – had resulted in a very low level of financial resources for public and private investment, according to the Ministry.

Macroeconomic policy was centred on the institutional and structural reform of the agricultural sector, the major source of economic growth (accounting for 70 per cent of GDP). In a nutshell, ending marketing monopolies and price controls, minimizing the trade bureaucracy, simplifying taxation, increasing and diversifying agricultural exports, and encouraging private investment were laid out as the main strategies for achieving continued strong growth, and the increase in import capacity through foreign exchange earnings to provide the basis for industrialization. Within this macroeconomic framework, sectoral spending on health and education was to be brought in line with the priorities of fiscal adjustment, including debt repayment. At the time, Uganda's debt burden was 56.9 per cent of exports and 3.4 per cent of GDP.[5] Basic health and education were acknowledged to be both human rights and important investments for the future productive capacity of the economy.[6] But in the context of 'severe resource constraints', the role of government, rather than 'heroically shouldering the entire burden of the health sector',[7] was to supervise the provision of health services – to establish a 'formal network in which NGO activities can be integrated to form a unified attack on the health problems in Uganda...the Government's role... to *guide* such a programme'.[8] In addition, the macroeconomic strategy specified that the limited public resources for the health sector should be concentrated on the provision of essential public goods (such as immunization, family planning, and AIDS education) as opposed to curative services. The strategy called for the establishment of private wings in government hospitals for those who 'wish to pay' related to their ability to pay. Health clinics, under the jurisdiction of District Councils were to introduce user fees to make up for revenue shortfalls. In addition to AIDS prevention, a comprehensive food and nutrition policy, and a national population programme, 'attempting to make population growth compatible with development in all parts of the country',[9] were laid out as the three specified targets of public health policy.

The Ugandan government's health policy framework mirrored the WB's framework of health expenditures and financing spelled out in the *Uganda Social Sector Strategy*, published in 1993. The Uganda policy framework was consistent with the WB's basic philosophy that the role of government should focus on three responsibilities: providing policy guidance, coordinating and monitoring the private sector and NGOs, and ensuring that government bureaucracy did not get in the way.[10] According to the strategy, certain services should remain the government's responsibility, defined as 'those which must be carried out by the government if they are to be provided in adequate quantities', such as health sector planning, education, basic sanitation, water, and environmental activities (although water privatization is on the current agenda). The second category of government involvement consisted of community health interventions of a preventive nature, such as vector control and vaccination. Curative services were to be primarily a private sector responsibility, and if the government was to provide curative care, it should do so by emulating the private sector, and should charge for them.[11]

Indeed, it was the case in Uganda in the early 1990s that the majority of public health expenditure was targeted at curative services – according to the WB, 90 per cent of health expenditure in 1992[12] – however, this was in a context of extremely inadequate spending in general. The public sector contributed approximately $2 per capita per annum to health, the lowest in the region. The 2000 figure has increased to $4, with private expenditure on health accounting for 62 per cent of all spending, 35 per cent of which is out of pocket, according to the WHO.[13] Shifting financing to PHC and prevention from curative services were to take place in a context where health care expenditure in general was woefully inadequate, the bulk of curative services already provided by the private sector. The logic of the shift according to the WB was that there would be little need for curative care if primary and preventative programmes were put in place. The spending devoted to curative care could be avoided through 'public action' such as AIDS education and nutritional counselling, the Social Sector Strategy maintained.[14] The WB's specific financing of AIDS prevention constituted such public action. AIDS prevention in the form of education, however, has had only partial relevance in parts of Uganda where HIV infection had peaked, where the sick have needed treatment and care, and where the survival of family members left behind was at stake.

The general path laid out in the early to mid-1990s has been followed, although the Ugandan government is considered to be driving the reform process. Christopher Adam argues that the Ugandan government has been in the driver's seat in determining macroeconomic policy reforms such as trade liberalization and exchange rate reform, and that it has been instrumental in designing the country's Poverty Eradication Action Plans (PEAP). He states that 'the Aid Liaison office [within the MFPED] circumscribes the role of donors: increasingly they are expected not to initiate and develop their own projects but to support activities identified, designed and implemented by the GOU'.[15] Uganda has been considered the IMF and the WB's 'Star Pupil' and has been held up as an example of success in sustaining high rates of economic growth through fiscal restraint and trade liberalization. Under the Heavily Indebted Poor Countries (HIPC) initiative, Uganda has obtained substantial debt relief and has been able to divert significantly more resources to health and education, poverty-related expenditures, increasing from approximately 18 per cent of the budget in the early 1990s to 35 per cent in 2002. But whether in the driver's seat or not, the 60 per cent fall in coffee prices that Uganda's liberalized economy has seen over the past few years has meant that the government had to borrow more to make up the shortfall. Uganda's debt to export ratio was 210 per cent in 2000–2001 and is projected to remain close to that level for the next few years.[16] It is also worth noting that donor assistance to Uganda equals 50 per cent of total government expenditure, roughly 10 per cent of GDP.[17] The room for the state to manoeuvre is to some degree circumscribed by the parameters established by donors and the WB, by debt repayment, as well as by the vagaries in global market prices for Uganda's export commodities.

The government's broad macropolicy agenda has remained relatively unchanged, despite the deep impact of HIV/AIDS-related mortality on productivity and household survival. AIDS policy and macroeconomic policy remain separate and distinct, despite the recognition, at least on paper, that the two are intertwined, as evidenced by a number of AIDS-impact assessments.[18] In the GOU *Strategies to Promote Economic Growth Progress Report*, the plan for the modernization of agriculture makes calls for a sustained increase in the productivity of agriculture, through increased privatization and commercialization, and makes no mention of HIV/AIDS, despite its negative impact on productivity and household food security. Calling on the one hand for 'pro-poor and gender-sensitive' policies, the report states that 'agricultural activity is a commercial activity, and such should be carried out by the private sector.'[19] A critical gap exists in understanding how particular policies and programmes have undermined rural livelihoods and food security in AIDS-afflicted communities. Growth in agricultural productivity can go hand in hand with increased household food insecurity and malnutrition in contexts where rural communities are heavily dependent on subsistence production alongside activity for the market. In SSA, women tend to produce food for household consumption and for local markets, while men tend to produce non-food commercial and export crops. What happens when their agricultural labour is diverted to caring for the sick, or when cash contributions to household income disappear on the death of their husband? In reality, macroeconomic policy development in general and agricultural policy in particular pay little heed to HIV/AIDS. It has been proven difficult to break out of the biomedical and public health boundaries of AIDS control and prevention.

The Uganda AIDS Control Programme

The formal institutional response to AIDS in Uganda began in October 1986 with the formation of the National Committee for the Prevention and Control of AIDS (NCPA) and the ACP; the advisory body and the executing body respectively, within the MOH. (The NCPA was collapsed into the ACP shortly after its formation.) The programme was conceived as one in which the MOH/ACP would provide technical leadership and coordination for all AIDS-related activities in the country. It was situated directly under the offices of the Minister of Health as a means of ensuring that resources would not be diverted to other programmes and that other important programmes in the Ministry would not be swallowed up by the ACP, however, the activities of the ACP were to be integrated into the PHC infrastructure and activities.[20] The response to AIDS in Uganda was part and parcel of the WHO's Global Programme, Uganda in fact the first recipient of a WHO-inspired and coordinated national programme. The programme followed WHO's 'Guidelines for the development of a national AIDS prevention and control programme'.[21] A director and a chief epidemiologist were appointed to oversee the four programme areas: epidemiology and research; IEC; laboratory/ blood transfusion; and clinical management, and a coordinator was assigned to each programme area. At the district level, District Medical Officers (DMOs) were in charge of ACP as part of their regular duties, and at the very local level the resistance committee chairman was given the responsibility of ensuring the success of the programme. All but two of the original eighteen appointees to the NCPA were medical professionals, the exceptions being a professor of sociology and a professor of social administration, both from Makerere University. Donor funds for the programme were to be coordinated by the WHO, and evaluations were to be carried out by the WHO Regional Office (WHO/AFRO) on a biannual basis. The initial short-term or emergency plan had as its stated objective 'the reduction of the spread of HIV virus and the reduction of the impact of the epidemic on communities, families and individuals'. The plan focused on basic medical interventions – making the case definition of AIDS available to public and private practitioners, conducting a national sample serosurvey, developing a surveillance system and an intensive system to screen blood transfusion products – interventions that were to be integrated into the existing health care system.

A more comprehensive and longer-term plan was developed with the WHO the following month, the 'ACP Proposals for a Five-Year Action Plan (1987–1991)', the result of a second WHO consultancy mission. The seven major components of the ACP were: mass public education and information; blood screening and rehabilitation of blood transfusion systems; protection of the public, health workers, and children through supply of syringes, needles, gloves, aprons, boots, disinfectants, equipment, condoms; establishment of an effective national surveillance system; drugs for treatment of AIDS cases; operational research consisting of KAP studies for health education, and sero-epidemiology and risk factors; and finally, training and orientation of health workers.[22] Technical and financial support provided by WHO and financial support from several donor agencies was coordinated by the ACP through the mechanism of a WHO trust fund. Funds were provided or committed to the trust by the UK, Sweden, USA, Denmark, Norway, and Italy, and from unspecified WHO global resources. In addition, bilateral support came from UNICEF, UNDP, the EEC, the Federal Republic of Germany, and USAID. The Ugandan government was to pay the recurrent costs of the programme – to provide office and physical facilities, pay salaries to staff at the district and local levels and pay maintenance expenses. The initial Five-year plan had a budget of just under US$7 million.

For purposes of discussion, the programme can be divided into two major components: first, clinical management and patient care; and second, behavioural interventions and education, although the two are not discrete categories and there is considerable overlap. The first component has consisted of rather standardized technical biomedical interventions such as cleaning up the blood supply, increasing resources for and developing protocols on patient care, and providing protective equipment to health care professionals. The second component has focused on 'education for behaviour change'. It would be a few years before the impact of the epidemic – already felt profoundly in the districts of highest concentration of infection – would be a concern of AIDS policy.

AIDS policy delivery: medical interventions

The deep crisis facing Uganda at the time of the appearance of HIV infection severely weakened precisely those government structures that were necessary for an effective response. A beleaguered MOH damaged by 20 years of civil war was given the task of containing the new epidemic. Health units, rural ones in particular, were derelict (lacking basics such as water and electricity) and poorly staffed. Health workers avoided postings to places where there was a lack of housing, schools, and other opportunities for income generation to supplement paltry government salaries. Staffing rural health units and dispensaries were nursing aides and dressers lacking in proper training. Basic drugs were supplied from 1985 onwards to all public clinics, hospitals, and NGO health units through Danish International Development Agency's (DANIDA) Basic Drugs Programme, but most drugs were either pilfered before arriving at the clinics or sold by underpaid health care staff through the private sector, a problem so acute that the DANIDA seriously considered the withdrawal of its support for the programme in 1992. Both lower-level and higher-level 'eating' was common. Budget allocations would disappear before meeting their final destination and health personnel would use the resources of the public system to bolster their private practices. The structural problems of health care delivery were reflected in the poor performance during the first few years of the ACP.

The original objective of the ACP Medium Term Plan with regard to patient care was 'to improve patient management' through a strategy of 'maintain[ing] optimal quality of life'.[23] The plan specified that patients being treated in government hospitals were to be referred to outpatient and/or traditional health care, rather than remain hospitalized during their illness. It was recommended that counselling of patients be provided, as part of both the initial inpatient treatment and the subsequent care for the patient in the home environment,[24] yet counsellors were few and far between. 'Outpatient care' was understood to be care in the extended family setting, and to this end the ACP recommended that small grants be made available to relatives of AIDS patients to cover extra expenses such as soap, other hygienic material, and herbal drugs,[25] although grants were never made available through the ACP. The vast majority of AIDS patients received no assistance whatsoever.

At the time the MTP was being formulated, there was an unpredicted steady rise in the number of AIDS patients in hospitals. In the major towns, 50 to 70 per cent of the adult inpatient hospital beds were occupied by patients with HIV-related illness by 1992.[26] In Jinja that same year, the only ward filled to capacity at the municipal hospital was the ward admitting AIDS patients.[27] The quality of patient care was hindered by extremely severe resource constraints, both financial and human. The ACP could not ensure the supply of the most basic of equipment to the public system to protect health workers and patients from HIV, such as protective gloves, gowns and masks, sterile needles, and soap. Also in short supply were basic antibiotics, antifungal, and antidiarrhoeal drugs to treat HIV-related opportunistic infections. Another documented problem was poor vehicle service and maintenance resulting in delays of quarterly drug-kit deliveries. And although sterilization equipment for reusable syringes was supplied to all hospitals and most health clinics, the electricity, required to run the equipment was sporadic. In units not serviced with electricity, there was often no kerosene to fuel the stoves for the steam sterilizers. The problems confronted were basic yet, in the context of such extreme resource shortages, seemed insurmountable to health care staff.

Given that hospital care was an area of health care provision where the private sector was expected to take on more responsibility, public spending on hospitals did not rise in response to the crisis in care created by rising numbers of HIV infected. Development assistance in the public sector increased, but most of the money at the time was earmarked for the rehabilitation of physical infrastructure. In any case, the majority of AIDS patients were being cared for outside the formal health system. Stated the 1991 ACP Plan and Budget: 'The reporting of AIDS cases who managed to get to a health facility leaves a lot to be desired; to this end the cumulative total of 17,422 AIDS cases as of 30 June 1990 is just a tip of the iceberg.'[28]

Blood transfusion services also fared poorly. Cleaning up the blood supply in Uganda was an obvious focus of the short-term and medium-term plan, as an estimated 8 per cent of infections were received through contaminated blood. A goal of the MTP was that 'at the end of twelve months new and existing blood transfusion centres should be fully equipped and running and all blood donations should be screened'.[29] In only one of the five regions constituting the Uganda Blood transfusion Service – the central region covering hospitals within a 100-km distance – was all blood tested for HIV and hepatitis in 1992. In 1991, WHO reported that blood transfusion continued to be a source of HIV infection, despite 4 years of sustained effort on the part of the WHO, the European Development Fund, the WB, and the Red Cross. It was still the case in 1992 that a guaranteed HIV-free unit of blood was not available in half the country's districts. Documented problems ranged from a shortage of trained staff and working vehicles to collect blood in the field and a shortage of cold storage facilities to handle supplies of blood, to banditry and break-ins at the centres. The recurrent costs of the MOH in meeting blood transfusion service requirements were difficult for the cash-strapped and resource-poor ministry to meet; at the same time, the donor community was not meeting its stated commitments. In 1991, the WHO/GPA in Uganda reported that:

> Inadequate, irregular and unpredictable mode of disbursement of funds from some donors meant that a lot of important blood transfusion objectives in peripheral areas could not be undertaken. Supervision of peripheral units was limited, supplies to these irregular, training was minimal and responsibility allowances were not paid in most cases resulting in poor performances.[30]

Donors withheld funds because they claimed that the spending of previous disbursements was unaccounted for. And indeed 'corruption' in the public health care system was a systemic problem. At a higher level, a number of WHO officials stated that budgetary allocations earmarked for specific purposes would often only partially be disbursed, the other part mysteriously disappearing. At the lower levels, the pilfering of funds might have had something to do with the fact that, at the time, stagnating civil service salaries barely covered the purchase of enough calories for three days for a family of four.[31] Requesting or extorting 'under-the-table' fees at government health units was a common practice, compounded by the bitterness of health staff at their inability to support their families on official salaries.[32] In this regard, the line between corruption and 'eating' was blurred; an extension of the logic of survival shaping everyday life for the majority of Ugandans.

The first few years of AIDS control in Uganda made clear that unless the infrastructure for basic health service provision throughout the country was sound, AIDS-specific programmes would perform poorly. Still, the trend is towards the establishment of vertical programmes, and increased emphasis on the privatization of services and cost recovery where it is deemed feasible. As the number of donor agencies mushroomed in the AIDS sector, the balance of activities shifted from activities under the direct control of the ACP towards semi-autonomous programmes and projects of the major donor institutions. The alternative to strengthening government health services was donor-funded projects filling in the gaps. All donors were required to meet the priorities as established by the ACP but in reality the MOH did not have the resources to monitor the growing number of AIDS projects.[33] A common complaint was the lack of remuneration to staff of the ACP. Staff would often not be at their desks, instead would be elsewhere engaged in other activities to supplement their salaries.

Given the poor state of the public health care system, the message of the WB/WHO/UNDP GOU mission of 1990 (which led to the Multisectoral AIDS Control Strategy) was that the provision of bilateral, private, NGO, and voluntary services and projects for AIDS patients must be strengthened. The WB emphasized the need for improving the administrative capacity of the state – stressing internal administrative efficiency and effectiveness – but at the same time called for the privatization of service delivery. The role of the state was to strengthen and support communities and families in providing care/counselling to AIDS patients. NGOs were providing alternatives to hospital-based care, although the demand for care greatly exceeded the supply. Most HIV-infected people were (and are still) cared for within their homes without public or private sector assistance, particularly in the rural areas. The 'core poor' simply do not have the resources to pay fees, whether formal or informal, or to pay for transport to the health centre. Privately run and church-based hospitals with external sources of funding were implementing mobile home-care programmes. One of the first was the RAIN which provided absolute basics such as aspirins, protective gloves, soap and bedding, as well as moral support to families who were caring for the diseased, and then burying their dead.

AIDS prevention: education for behaviour change

The 'ultimate goal' of the research component of the ACP in Uganda was to aid in the discovery of a vaccine or cure, but until that time the only way to halt progression of HIV infection was through behaviour change, in essence, through promoting monogamy, 'stable polygamy', or safer sex. Condom use was at the beginning a contentious issue, but by the 1990s was quietly promoted, although the Pope's visit in 1993 represented a major setback when he openly condemned condom use and preached that chastity and monogamy were the only solutions to the AIDS scourge. Considered by policy-makers to be at the root of the presumably high levels of promiscuity was modernization and urbanization, resulting in the breakdown of traditional cultural and moral codes that governed sexual relations.

Underlying the main accounts of risk behaviour was a reified notion of 'culture' removed from space and time, which constituted an explanation not only for rapid HIV and STD spread, but for the masking of the political and economic realities that shaped the specific Ugandan context of HIV spread: labour migration, continued instability, and particularly for women, insecurity of land tenure, and men's control of their sexuality and production.

The first educational interventions were mass-media activities – billboards, posters, pamphlets, and radio and newspaper advertisement – warning people to 'love carefully' and 'zero graze', and imparting information about the main transmission routes. AIDS awareness throughout the country was almost universal by 1990. In this regard, the first decade of AIDS control had a positive impact. But the ACP admitted in 1992 that its mass education campaigns had not sustained changes in 'high-risk' behaviour throughout the general population, stating that '...IEC activities have resulted in a very high level of HIV/ AIDS awareness nationally. This level of awareness has apparently not, however, been matched by an equally significant change in high-risk sexual behaviour.'[34] Evidence pointed to resistance to abstinence and monogamy as practical or realistic behavioural options. 'The major finding from this study is the importance of sexuality in everyday Ugandan life...shown in varied ways including frequency of multiple sexual partners and contacts that people have now, or have had in the past.'[35] 'Education for behaviour change' became the main locus of intervention. Just less than 27 per cent of the 1991 budget for the ACP was targeted at AIDS education. There were a variety of approaches to achieving the common goal; some such as USAID-favoured vertical, individual behaviour-oriented programmes involving condom promotion and distribution, and treatment of sexually transmitted infections (STIs), while others emphasized 'community-based' approaches which integrated other aspects of AIDS prevention and care (such as income generation and mobile home care). NGOs were to be instrumental in getting the message across and providing services.

Supplementing the activities of the ACP were the programmes of the most important international donor institutions: UNICEF, USAID, CARE, MSF, GTZ, Save the Children, and AMREF. USAID was the largest single player in AIDS education through its AIDSCOM projects, as well as a whole range of projects executed through the US-based

NGO 'Experiment in International Living', and supported the activities of the ACP. Donors have had considerable freedom to design their interventions at arms length from the MOH and the ACP. USAID channelled most of its funding through AIDSCOM – a public health communication programme administered by the US-based Academy for Educational Development aligned with US-based consulting groups which carried out the planning, monitoring, and evaluation of AIDSCOM projects. A central component of AIDSCOM's 'Public Health Communication Support Program' consisted of training peer educators and trainers in the workplace, who would in turn communicate messages to co-workers and act as role models for behaviour change. It was predominantly urban men of high educational level who were exposed to the programme in a workplace setting. A similar programme had reached 53 NGOs through AIDSCOM's technical assistance to the US-based NGO, Experiment in International Living (now called World Learning).

According to their programme evaluations, there was no significant visible change in number of sexual partners, although there was a marginal increase in condom use. The programme, however, was considered a success because 'indicators of programme activity show that the programme has been implemented successfully, with significant increases in the number who report talking to a peer educator, attending a talk about AIDS in the workplace, and seeing the dramatic film "Its Not Easy" '.[36] The quantitative indicators of programme evaluation were such that as long as the programme was smoothly implemented, it was deemed successful. By focusing on well-educated urban males and condom use as the main strategy of HIV prevention, USAID was able to sidestep the more thorny issues relating to the socio-economic and cultural barriers to safe sex which were encountered by a large section of the female population and the rural poor. The same can be said of its vertical, STD control projects. USAID also funded the $15 million 'STD Prevention and Control Project', its purpose was to limit the impact of HIV/AIDS infection in 'target populations' through interventions that promote changes in sexual behaviours and reduce risk factors, in this case, sexually transmitted infections.

An important component of the STDCP was the pilot research project CHIPS – 'Community Health Intervention Project against STDs' – implemented in Kisenyi, a densely populated, low-income neighbourhood in Kampala. It was a comprehensive set of activities including testing, treatment, and counselling for STIs, and community health initiatives including condom promotion and peer education. The main objective of the project was to reduce the spread of HIV in the community through the treatment of STIs and to determine the best way to go about STI control. According to the head of STD control in the MOH, CHIPS was the only comprehensive project of its kind in the country. Some of the insights from CHIPS were raised by the chief investigator on the project, a physician from the University of California, at the Post-Amsterdam Public Seminar of Uganda-based AIDS Researchers organized by the UAC in October 1992. Cheryl Walker found that counselling of individuals was of limited success and that condom use was not consistently effective because it was not female-controlled. Given the stigma and shame attached to STIs, women in particular were not attending clinics. Walker's comments spoke about the limitations of vertical interventions that focused on individual behaviour and STI treatment without regard for the specific social conditions that influenced access to and use of services, and the ability to adopt less risky behaviours, such factors as the lack of privacy and visibility within the community in a context where women were largely blamed for the spread of infection. Significant stigma was attached to attending the STD clinic, more so for women than for men. And it was not the case that all women could negotiate condom use.

Walker was aware of the limitations of the project and sought to introduce different approaches. She viewed enhancing women's negotiating skills through community-based organizing and couples counselling as more promising options to the current approach of individual counselling. But women's power in negotiating sex was and is not simply a matter of 'skill' and empowerment. Women's unequal power in intimate relationships was related to the pervasive view of sex within marriage for women as a marital obligation, and the view that married women and their labour are the physical property of their husbands. Some women acquiesced in unwanted sex for fear of being abandoned or stripped of their means of support.

The largest project under the control of the ACP, the District AIDS Mobilization Project (DAMP), went beyond individual counselling and condom promotion. The DAMP was a project designed by the Health Education Division of the MOH in collaboration with the ACP and began after a programme review of the ACP's AIDS education and prevention activities in 1988. Prior to 1988, prevention activities were limited to Kampala, but by 1992 20 of Uganda's 38 districts had DAMP. Plans were developed by the ACP in collaboration with the DMO in each district, and were geared towards the use of existing structures at the district level: health staff, local-level RCs, NGOs, and religious groups. The programme's implementation was constrained by the same structural factors, that limited the success of other components of the ACP related to the lack of funds and weak institutional capacity: 'at a technical level Damp was never provided with the financial nor the central infrastructural resources to fulfil its mandate'.[37] Further,

> it seems that in planning DAMP activities there was over-expectation of time and resources available to the RC system in this case, for AIDS education. In particular, there was strong evidence that the district department heads had not the time, and perhaps not the inclination, to be actively involved in AIDS education.[38]

Programme activities included the reproduction of AIDS educational materials in the form of booklets, pamphlets, and posters on AIDS, training seminars for health workers, government administrators, and NGO representatives, and a mass campaign on prevention and control. The general public was expected to receive materials through the LCs and key people such as mass mobilizers and development workers in the community. The main strategies to control the spread of AIDS included abstinence, monogamy, and the promotion of alternate recreational activities. An evaluation of the DAMP was conducted between July and December 1991. Three districts were chosen for the evaluation: one with no DAMP, one where DAMP had been ongoing, and one with recent DAMP. A key finding of the evaluation: 'There appears to be little difference in awareness to AIDS and knowledge about the basic facts about AIDS between the two districts that have DAMP compared to Mbale which does not.'[39] Among the sample, knowledge of the sexual transmission of AIDS was high, at 99 per cent in all three districts. But there was no related evidence of sustained sexual behaviour change across the sample population. Nor was there evidence of alternative income generating and recreational activities despite their encouragement, this latter point reminding me of the laughter met by the slogan 'don't play sex, rebuild your country' by some young people in Jinja in the context of a casual discussion about AIDS at a community meeting. These are the words of a 20-year-old man:

> What else are we to do here, when after 7 o'clock there is no light and unlike you, we have no TV's or places to go? Instead of enjoying ourselves, they want us to fill up the pot holes in the roads.[40]

In 1992, UNICEF introduced SYFA, 'Safeguarding Youth from AIDS'. SYFA attributed the failure of message-based campaigns providing AIDS strategies on the messages themselves – they called for monogamy among populations whose sexual behaviour was already established as non-monogamous, they were negative and relied on fear, and they failed to target pre-sexually active youth. The basic assumption was that the AIDS epidemic could begin to be brought under control in a measurable way within 5 years as the 9–14-year-olds who were free of the virus moved into the more sexually active 15–19-year cohort and beyond. SYFA would meet its measurable targets by empowering youth – especially girls – to make informed decisions based on a set of plausible alternative behaviours: the delay of sexual debut; celibacy and abstinence; faithful monogamous relationships; and the practice of safer sex including the correct and regular use of condoms. If learned at an early age, these behaviours might be maintained in adulthood. SYFA was implemented through established channels: NGOs, churches, and the RCs, as well as through UNICEF's School Health Education Project. A key component of the project was to assist national and local capacity to make the programme sustainable. An evaluation of the programme conducted in 1995 pointed to the difficulties, both in achieving targets and in fostering local sustainability. Most of the problems were related to the poor institutional abilities of the executing organizations and the very low levels of funding, often far below what was needed to implement their programmes; other problems reflected local struggles for power and resources. HIV rates have dropped among this cohort, although remain higher for girls.

Despite the fact that AIDS education was reportedly not resulting in widespread behaviour change, levels of HIV seroprevalence began to drop. How do we explain the drop, given the reports on marginal changes in sexual behaviour, and the widespread and systemic problems of the implementation of the ACP on the ground? Helen Epstein questions whether the epidemic is truly waning; pointing out that the incidence of infection – the rate at which people become infected – may be stable or even rising in some areas, while the prevalence – the number of infected people in a population – is falling. She points to smaller studies conducted by epidemiologists that show little change in incidence throughout the 1990s. Epstein hypothesizes that the first phase of HIV infection likely resulted from 'one-off' sexual encounters during the war, a time in which high numbers of soldiers carried HIV, rape was very common, and women in areas of the highest concentration of infection were drawn into sexual servicing out of economic necessity.[41]

> The hypothesis that the HIV epidemic in Uganda occurred in two phases implies that HIV prevalence may have fallen in the 1990s because many people infected during the war in the 1980s died of AIDS. Nevertheless, HIV incidence rates during peace-time may still be quite high, although they are probably much lower than they were during the war.[42]

Likely the ACP also contributed to declining rates of infection, but the extent to which AIDS education has contributed to declines in infection remains an open question. But what the policy response was not addressing was the effects and impacts of AIDS outside the health care sector – hence the emergence of the multisectoral strategy. As the first articulation of the Multisectoral Approach stated, 'the HIV/AIDS epidemic has produced socio-cultural, psychological, economic, moral, ethical, and legal ramifications, each with current or potentially catastrophic implications, and issues that the health sector has never been equipped to handle'.[43]

The multisectoral strategy

The formulation of Uganda's multisectoral strategy for AIDS reflected the evolution of thinking within the international AIDS community more generally, which by the early 1990s was increasingly viewing the epidemics in Africa as a concern beyond the health sector. It also corresponded to the emergence of UNAIDS. The document *AIDS Control in Uganda: The Multisectoral Approach* provides the following rationale for broadening the scope and mandate for AIDS control and prevention:

> Coordination efforts of the Ministry of Health ACP helped to create the high national level of awareness about the disease that now exists. The programme also played an important role in bringing the international community to the assistance of Uganda. However, coordination of activities being in the health sector, the epidemic continued to be addressed as primarily a health problem. Consequently, there has been limited response by the public sectors of information, labour, local administration, and youth and culture. The social and economic implications of the epidemic have not, therefore, received as much vigorous attention as they should.[44]

The UAC was formed to play an 'enabling role' in all national efforts. Under the umbrella of the Commission, all AIDS control interventions in the public and private sectors would be planned, implemented, budgeted for, and evaluated.[45] The multisectoral strategy corresponded to the WB's more authoritative voice in health policy, both within UNAIDS and in Uganda specifically. The WB was the largest single donor to the multisectoral strategy.[46] The total budget of the UAC was estimated at US$4,427,000, of which slightly less than half had been pledged by 1993. The GOU was the main funder of the UAC, but in 1993, USAID, through World Learning, was paying the salaries of the secretariat, which were high compared to other government employees. It was unclear what the relationship would be between the highly paid UAC and the struggling MOH ACP, the politics between the two described as extremely difficult by more than one senior policy official with USAID. But the structural contradiction of a well-funded bureaucracy financed with outside monies overseeing the activities of the poorly financed health sector, NGOs, and CBOs was bound to create tensions.

The role of the UAC was to guide and monitor the activities of the other ministries, the charitable and the private sectors, in line with broader policy reforms taking place at both national and local levels. 'One of the key assumptions was that on-going policy reforms would continue in favour of strengthening the role of women in development (WID), decentralization of planning and service provision, promotion of self-reliance and community empowerment, and developing close partnership between government, NGOs and CBOs.'[47] Thus began the development of a Kampala-based bureaucracy to guide community-based district level interventions and to 'empower' people to cope.

The goals and strategies of the Multisectoral AIDS Approach were stated as follows: to stop the spread of HIV infection; to mitigate the adverse health and socio-economic impact of the HIV/AIDS epidemic; to strengthen national capacity to respond to the HIV/AIDS epidemic; to establish a national information base on HIV/AIDS; and to strengthen the national capacity to undertake research relevant to HIV/AIDS.[48] *The Uganda National Operational Plan for HIV/AIDS/STD Prevention, Care and Support 1994–1998*, the outcome of the National AIDS Consensus Conference, and the National AIDS Planning Workshop held in Kampala in June 1993 were the first steps in operationalizing the strategy. The Ministry of Local Government was given the responsibility of coordination at the district level, in line with the government's decentralization policies. The implementation of the various components of the strategy was earmarked as the responsibility of local and foreign-based NGOs, local level committees, and the private sector, including traditional healers, and individuals and families. The wisdom of how to prevent transmission of HIV (as well as other STIs) had evolved from a strict focus on individual behaviour change, given the wide 'knowledge vs. moral behaviour change gap'[49] throughout the country.

To address the behaviours, practices and other factors determining the sexual transmission of HIV infection it is not sufficient to address the individual's behaviours only, as these are to a very great extent determined by factors over which the individual has limited control. The priorities of the programme over the next five years therefore, will focus on empowering the individual and at the same time addressing norms, values and collective behaviours and practices.[50]

To this end, three main areas were selected as priorities: first, children and youth; second, 'gender issues and the special situation and needs of women, particularly rural women and occupationally pre-disposed and exposed women – barmaids, prostitutes, clerical workers and house girls'; and third, 'situations and sites – the places and events where increased risk of sexual transmission occurs, such as visits to bars, discos and social functions, last funeral rites, weddings, twin ceremonies, offices, truck stops, migrant work situation, offices, factories'.[51] Within all government ministries, AIDS-related sectoral policies were to be developed, and all ministries were expected to establish ACP in their specific sectors – Defence, Education, Information, Labour and Social Affairs, and Local Government. So, for example, the MOH was to oversee AIDS surveillance, safe blood, and IEC; the Ministry of Labour was charged with developing policy guidelines for NGOs, private charities, and local communities for orphans and other children, and assessing the impact of changing demographics; the Ministry of Defence was to improve condom use, HIV testing, counselling, family planning, and care of HIV-infected soldiers, in addition to assessing the impact of the epidemic on the military.[52]

The second goal of the multisectoral strategy was to mitigate the socio-economic impact, although UAC acknowledged difficulty in this regard from the beginning. The impediments to mitigation activities were not only the thin knowledge base – very few specific studies on the impact of HIV/AIDS have yet been carried out – but also the lack of financial resources, in particular the deficit that in the words of the UAC 'hinders rational planning'.[53] At the time (between 1995 and 1996), the government was transferring approximately US$200 million to the IMF as part of the debt service of Uganda's US$3.1 billion debt it owed to the institution and other bilateral donors.[54] What was clear was that the National Operational Plan would target 'the individual and family in the community at the grassroots level'.[55] One half of the overall proposed budget was earmarked for mitigating the impact – US$246 million over the four-year period, over half of this sum was allotted specifically for orphans.[56] With regard to orphan support, the public sector's role was to develop standards of community-based care and education, solicit funds, strengthen welfare offices, promote awareness of possible neglect of fostered children, and to monitor the adherence to the rules and policy guidelines for the care of orphans.[57] The anticipated impact of AIDS on various sectors was delineated in brief (agriculture, industry, transport and communication, health, education, public administration, and national security) and viewed principally in terms of impact on the labour supply and productivity, as well as on public expenditures, and private investment and savings. Suggestions as to what 'could be done' were briefly summarized. For example in agriculture, the recommended interventions included the introduction of more appropriate and affordable means of production (for example, labour-saving technologies and high yielding, early maturing and resistant crop varieties), the improvement in research and training methods, and enhanced credit provision and marketing.[58]

How these policy goals were to be implemented was not spelled out in the operational plan, and with the exception of orphan support, were not translated into concrete policy. In 2000, a new National Strategic Framework for HIV/AIDS Activities was designed by a core group of 11 stakeholders from the UAC, MOH, Local Government, MFPED, and other organizations working in the AIDS sector and PLWAs, organized around the themes of prevention, care, mitigation and research.[59] The framework placed more emphasis on mitigation, and specified what was involved, but left untouched a consideration of the relationship between macroeconomics and HIV/AIDS. The current discourse on 'community', 'partnership', 'ownership', and 'empowerment' is used to articulate an approach to mitigation that is unquestioning of the neoliberal framework within which communities are to cope with the impacts of AIDS morbidity and mortality.

The community response

What community means in the multisectoral strategy is broad. LCs are the geographic and political units responsible for overseeing the implementation of the multisectoral strategy, as are local and northern-based NGOs, private health practitioners, traditional healers and birth attendants, church-based organizations, and individuals and families. Women are singled out for specific consideration – previously the invisible farmers, they are now the visible nurses of HIV sufferers who need to be encouraged and 'empowered' in their new role. The multisectoral strategy states that '...communities which have been sensitized about their own role in the management of HIV/AIDS will need to identify local sources of support (financial, material, spiritual) that will enable them to take full responsibility for their sick'.[60] What is implied is that within the broad managerial frame of AIDS control and prevention, targeted interventions can empower individuals and local groups to deal with the AIDS crisis, while at the same time tapping into local knowledges and capacities, and fostering self-reliance.

Communities were struggling with the effects of HIV/AIDS as early as the late 1980s. An enumeration and needs assessment of orphans carried out in 1989 documented the increasing pressure being experienced by extended family systems due to the demographic damage caused by high AIDS mortality. The large number of children orphaned in the wars since 1971 had mostly been absorbed through fostering systems and family networks. But in the context of the near complete breakdown in essential services coupled with increasing numbers of orphans due to AIDS, the ability of the 'extended family' to care for orphans was crumbling. In 1989, 12.8 per cent of children in the district of Rakai had been orphaned. The definition of 'orphan' for the purposes of the enumeration was a child who had lost only one parent. In the case of the father's death, this definition makes more sense, because in the majority of cases where the father dies, the mother is no longer the child's guardian, the responsibility shifting to the father's clan. Children whose parents had both died of AIDS were considered the worst off, followed by children whose father had died of AIDS. In the event of a husband's death, women would often be chased off their husband's land by their husband's clansmen and would take the smallest child or children who were still being breastfed, and would seek out remarriage, or some existence in Kampala. The older children would stay behind, cared for by women of the father's clan. It was reported that widows who did stay behind to care for their children could not expect any assistance from her husband's relatives, and had no say in clan decisions. Often they were allotted a plot too small to grow enough food, making their burden overwhelming.[61]

Janet Seeley and others conducted a study during the period January–June 1991 on 30 clients of the counselling component of the MRC Programme on AIDS in Uganda, who had requested home-based care. The objective of the study was to assess the family response to coping with the care of AIDS patients, given the commonly held assumption of policy-makers that the extended family system is a national strength in the context of AIDS care and prevention. Their findings suggested that the care of AIDS patients in the community often fell on individuals with limited assistance from extended kin. There were a number of reasons given why the care given by caregivers often fell short in some way, including lack of food in the home, lack of money for medications, and other responsibilities including the care of children, cultivation, care of other sick relatives; care was also denied because of stigma and blame. The following case was offered as the typical experience of a poor, AIDS-infected household:

> [The client]...was a 35 year old woman whose husband had died earlier in the year. She was living close to her elderly mother-in-law, who was too weak to help. She had seven children. The youngest two aged three and six months were sick. Her son aged 16 and daughter aged 15 cared for their mother. On two occasions the eldest son went to fetch his maternal grandmother, who lived some distance away, when he believed his mother to be dying. On both occasions this proved not to be the case, the grandmother returned to her own home because of her own family responsibilities. When the client died the extended family gathered for the funeral, but returned to their homes after the funeral rites leaving behind the 16 year old boy as household head in charge of his six siblings.[62]

In 1992, I met with a number of people living in AIDS-afflicted households in Kampala, Jinja, and the surrounding rural regions. Not untypical was a 50-year-old female craft seller in Kampala, divorced, with five children and three grandchildren. Only her youngest daughter was living with her when her eldest son came home to die. She was supporting her son and two grandchildren with no other support from 'extended kin'. To supplement her income, she grew beans, cassava, and matooke on an empty plot of land near her house. When asked about extended kin, she stated that two of her daughters are unemployed and have nothing to share. Her other son was not interested, having his own child to take care of. 'These days in Kampala, we take care of ourselves' were her words.[63] Another example: a young woman infected with HIV living with her infant and toddler and her aging mother in a hut on municipal land, who survived by growing potatoes and groundnuts, and collecting wild mangoes and greens. Her mother was too old to work, but would be left with the children if they survived – both were malnourished and sickly. This woman had knowledge about HIV/AIDS transmission, but said that she would have sex with any man if he helped support her and her children. She has not been targeted by any HIV/AIDS interventions.

There is great variation in community-based AIDS-related activities in Uganda. On one end of the spectrum are groups of widows securing small grants or microloans to start a piggery- or poultry-raising project for the raising of school fees; often these groups falter as quickly as they are formed. (A women's group in Jinja that had secured a small amount of funding from UK-based charity collapsed when the piglets purchased escaped from their pen – they did not know how they would pay back the loan.) On the other end is an organization like TASO, which commands hundreds of thousands of dollars and has an international reputation. Many of the local agencies, whether small or large, receive funding and technical assistance from foreign or international NGOs operating within Uganda's borders – such as MSF, Care, Save the Children, AMREF, Canadian Physicians for Aid and Relief, Concern, World Vision, the Christian Children's Fund, and Oxfam, whose activities in most cases pre-date the AIDS epidemic. The boundaries between the community, northern NGOs and the state are blurred, even to the extent that in some cases NGOs are contributing to the operating budgets of government departments.

The first indigenous AIDS-specific NGO in the AIDS sector was TASO founded in 1987. TASO became the model for other NGOs involved in patient care in the country and in the region, and quickly developed an international reputation. TASO assists families in the care of sick relatives through the provision of information and counselling, food, some clinical support, and home-care kits containing items such as protective gloves, soap, and antiseptic creams. In 1993, it had branches in eight districts, and mobile home programmes within a 20-mile radius of its offices. TASO also provides 'encouragement' for income-generating activities among families in order to alleviate their economic problems, although its activities in this regard are limited. The main focus of TASO's activities has been emotional support, education, and clinical care. Anthony Klouda observed in 1992 that NGO reliance upon external donor funding to provide services that the public sector was not equipped to provide was beginning to breed distortion in the provision of health services, TASO was receiving so much funding that it could provide comprehensive health and social support service for people with HIV. But the problem was that no equivalent existed for people with other very serious health problems (the public service paled in comparison) and that its reach was limited.[64]

TASO's very good services can be contrasted with those available in the southwestern district of Kisoro. The AIDS Programme of St Francis Hospital, called the Hope Clinic, was one of the few programmes in Kisoro District in 1995. Sub-clinics at the parish level did not exist and for some patients it was four hours walk to the clinic, which was held every Wednesday, when food and treatment were made available free of charge. The clinic had other programmes as well, providing support for orphans, client-group counselling, a home-visitor's programme, and support for income generation. A study of the services was carried out between 1995 and 1996. Thirty people associated with the Hope Clinic who were affected by AIDS were followed – clients, orphans, and their guardians. The findings were taken as the basis for five main recommendations to improve the programme, which involved increasing the cultural, economic, and social capital of clients. To summarize, five main directives were proposed: (1) education, training, and seminars to make clients aware that AIDS-related issues should be put in place; (2) clients should be supported to set up income generation; (3) clients should be stimulated to be involved in social groups; (4) communities should be made to share the responsibility for clients in the villages; and (5) more initiatives should be developed to reach unregistered AIDS patients in the district.[65]

In Kisoro District, self-reliance was taken to a new level. The problems and recommendations reflect the degree to which AIDS patients and their families are left to fend for themselves. Avoiding dependence and creating responsibility were emphasized. Clients of the clinic – the ones who are still physically strong enough – were the volunteers for the home-visitor's programme. The initiative was not functioning very well because 'clients raise their hands when they are asked to join the home visitor team, but they never show up'.[66] To help this component of the programme succeed better, the report suggests that volunteers could be trained and given a certificate stating that they are qualified to administer basic drugs. In addition, home visitors could be stimulated more by giving them free food in the clinic or a T-shirt after finishing the training seminar. It was also recommended that to increase their economic capital, clients (be they HIV positive, suffering from AIDS, or caring for one or more sick family members at home) propose a sustainable plan for income generation, for which loans should be made available (rather than grants, which foster dependency), such as a credit and savings group or rotating funds.[67] This begs the question of who is to pay off the loan once the client is dead, a serious problem when it means that when assets such as land or profits are taken over, the spouse or children are saddled with repayment or the loan is written off, creating strain for the creditor. The author points to the specific difficulties of setting income-generating projects in Kisoro District: 'lack of education, overpopulation, shortage of land, lack of running water, bad roads, etcetera'.[68] Moreover, 'most clients do not have a long future anymore and their needs are urgent. This requires income generating activities that can make a fast profit'.[69] It is suggested that the clinic could organize workshops, having positive effects on coping behaviour; needlework, mat weaving, table-cloth making, repairing second-hand clothes. The report acknowledges that certain people might not be available for income generation – for instance, widows supporting children on a subsistence basis – in short, those most marginalized and in need of assistance. The programme has a structure similar to TASO's, which in turn was modelled on the ASOs that sprung up in the affluent gay communities in Europe and North America. The meaning of empowerment and self-reliance in the context of deep economic crisis and social marginalization, where everyday life is a struggle for survival, HIV notwithstanding, takes on a more sinister connotation. Weaving mats and baskets in order to pay for one's funeral is perhaps the ultimate expression of self-reliance.

The local NGOs that do manage to secure funding through northern NGOs often can provide services beyond the scope of the Hope Clinic in Kisoro. More than 700 agencies in Uganda are involved in direct service delivery to the community in 2001, according to a survey conducted by AMREF and commissioned by the UAC. In such a context, despite the fact that through the UAC the control of AIDS policy is in Ugandan hands, it is very difficult to imagine that programmes can be evenly distributed, can be 'unified' and 'integrated' into the overall policy response, and that the limited resources that do exist are being used in the most 'cost-effective' and 'efficient' manner. While local NGOs and CBOs compete with each other for project funding, few question why there are no resources for increased public spending in the health and social sectors. Hence the reliance on 'the community' – essentially women's unpaid labour – onto whom contradictions and wider problems can be offloaded. This is not to denigrate the very real efforts of NGOs and community groups working on the margins, nor is it to say that their interventions have no impact. Indigenous NGOs such as Ugandan Women's Effort to Save the Orphans (UWESO), made up largely of female volunteers established before the HIV/AIDS epidemic in response to the problem of children orphaned during the war, has 35 branches and assist communities to support orphans; Uganda Community-based Association for Child Welfare (UCOBAC) is a network similar to UWESO with a focus on sustainable 'community-based' initiatives, education, and income generation targeted largely at women who are caring for the current one in nine children who are orphans across the country. These organizations, and ones like them, provide much-needed care to the most vulnerable. But it is the case that wider constraints, embodied in the relationship between donors, the local and central government and financial institutions, and the fragile and impoverished nature of communities, limit the scope of AIDS-specific interventions.

The National Strategic Framework for HIV/AIDS Activities, which was drawn up to cover the period 1998–2002, placed more emphasis on the specifics of mitigation at the individual, household, and community levels, and has called for the expansion of microcredit and income generation as solutions to economic impacts at the household level. 'Support to people with AIDS to start up income generating projects is extremely essential...but should be monitored consistently to limit mismanagement and capital loss.'[70] The 'community' is to be supported through income-generating projects, and the private sector is to be mobilized to provide more resources to support people living with AIDS. Palliative care is to be strengthened through the provision of training for people in the home, traditional healers, and religious leaders, and subsidies are to be granted for the treatment of opportunistic infections. Financial support is to be extended for child-headed households and AIDS orphans.

Few AIDS-related interventions have been established outside the parameters of health education, orphan care, and fostering self-sufficiency. In response to the growing problem of widows being chased off of their land, or their children being taken on the event of their husband's death, The Uganda Women Lawyer's Association (FIDA) instituted legal aid clinics in urban and rural centres for women without access to a lawyer, and has held seminars to teach, interpret, and discuss the laws of Uganda having to do with land, inheritance, and children, at local community schools. They have translated the law pertaining to women's rights into local languages and have lobbied for amendments to several existing laws, particularly the succession and inheritance laws that are unfair to women.

Those within the AIDS community in Uganda, who are involved on the ground, struggle with the constraints imposed by the funding institutions, by a weak state with few financial resources, and by the specific local conditions that shape survival strategies in the hardest-hit communities. Joyce Butera, a counsellor with the Rakai project, said that people's daily struggles to survive mean that they do not have time to think about AIDS. The Project Manager of World Learning's AIDS Prevention and Control project said that donor staff were aware that their interventions are essentially microsolutions to what are macroproblems, and that the very structure of development assistance militated against institutional capacity-building and 'ownership' of projects by the stakeholders. 'We have no desire to perpetuate ourselves, but what can we do in what is essentially an emergency situation?' He also pointed out that the NGOs themselves are beholden to their funders. 'USAID regulations are extremely constraining, and simply getting approval and authorization is a bureaucratic nightmare.'[71]

It is in this context that new partnerships are being developed to 'scale up' ARV access in Uganda. In August 2003, the Director of Health Services announced that all Ugandans suffering from AIDS would have access to free ARVs. The MOH was preparing to buy the drugs with resources from the Global Health Fund, and the ACP was working out the details for delivering treatment.[72] The number given for those in immediate need of treatment was stated to be 150,000 among the 1.2 million infected people. Uganda had reached agreements with four of the main pharmaceutical companies in 2000 for substantial price cuts, under the four-country pilot project spearheaded by UNAIDS, the HIV/AIDS Drugs Access Initiative. Launched in partnership with the Ugandan MOH, the pilot project has involved training and capacity building at six regional hospitals to provide access to ARV treatment at cost. Prices have been in the neighbourhood of about $250 a month for double therapy and $420 for triple therapy, although prices have fluctuated – rapid currency devaluation resulting at one point in an increase of 20 per cent of the cost to patients.[73] The pilot project has proven that some Ugandans can benefit from ARV treatment. But the cost of a month's drugs is far beyond the reach of the vast majority of Ugandans, and given the current state of the health care system, there is deep scepticism about how the public provision of ARVs will ever be realized. Who will get access to treatment, and who will fall through the cracks? How can all Ugandans in need receive ARVs when half the population still lacks access to the very basics, when outpatient health care is free only in principle, when money for transport is still a major impediment to seeking health care, when there is still a chronic shortage of trained health personnel? When, according to the National Strategic Framework 1998–2002, condoms are still inaccessible and unaffordable to the majority of people, voluntary counselling and testing services exist only in 31 out of 56 districts, there are no staff and rooms to provide counselling in hospitals, and laboratories lack inputs?[74]

The major constraints on HIV/AIDS programme implementation were captured and summarized by AMREF in its survey of agencies working in the AIDS sector.

> Most agencies have been unable to break the vicious cycle of poverty that propels the spread of HIV infection, precipitates the development of AIDS, compounds its psycho-social impact on the affected, and negatively impacts on the quality of life for PLWA, eventually reducing the productive potential of the affected in the community. Companion to this problem are the high illiteracy rate, gender inequality, sex discrimination, stereotyped attitudes and traditional practices that negatively impact on one's rights and individuality.[75]

Nelson Sewankambo, a medical doctor aligned with a number of AIDS projects, echoed these sentiments back in 1992. 'The biggest impediment to the local response is the vicious circle of poverty that is unending. We don't have time to look at the bigger picture ... we can't afford to look at the bigger picture.'[76]

Notes

1. UNDP, *Human Development Report 2003* (New York: Oxford University Press, 2003) 246.
2. UNAIDS/UNICEF/WHO, 'Epidemiological Fact Sheet on HIV/AIDS and STIs', Update (Uganda, 2002) 2.
3. Human Rights Watch, 'Just Die Quietly: Domestic Violence and Women's Vulnerability to HIV', *Human Rights Watch Report* 15.15(a) (Aug. 2003): 2.
4. Uganda Ministry of Planning and Economic Development (UMPED), *The Way Forward I: Macroeconomic Strategy 1990–1995 and the Way Forward II: Medium Term Sectoral Strategy 1991–1995* (Entebbe: Government Printers, Jan. 1992) i.
5. UNDP, 293.
6. UMPED, 34–36.
7. Ibid., 36.
8. Ibid., 37.
9. Ibid., 37.
10. World Bank, *Uganda: Growing Out of Poverty* (Washington, D.C.: World Bank, 1993) 119.
11. Ibid., *Uganda Social Sector Strategy* (1993).
12. Ibid., *Growing*, 111.
13. WHO, 'Selected health indicators for Uganda' (http://www3.who.int/whosis/country/indicators.cfm?country=uga&language=en).
14. World Bank, *Social Sector*, 67.
15. Christopher Adam, 'Redesigning the Aid Contract: Donors' Use of Performance Indicators in Uganda', *World Development*, 30 (Dec. 2002): 2046.
16. Romilly Greenhill, 'New World Bank Reports Confirm that HIPC Initiative is Failing', *Jubilee Research* (29 Apr. 2002) 4.
17. Adam, 2049.
18. See, for example, Tony Barnett and Alan Whiteside, 'The Social and Economic Impact of HIV/AIDS in Poor Countries: A Review of Standards and Practices', *Progress in Development Studies* 1.2 (2001): 151–70; Lori Bollinger, John Stover, and Vastha Kibirige, 'The Economic Impact of AIDS in Uganda', unpublished paper, Futures Group International (Sept. 1999); Daphne Topouzis, 'Uganda: The Socio-economic Impact of HIV/AIDS on Rural Families with an Emphasis on Youth' (Rome: FAO, Feb. 1994).
19. GOU, *Strategies to Promote Economic Growth Progress Report* (Kampala, May 2003) 5 (http://www.worldbank.org/ug/cg03/CG_2003_GoU_Growth_Paper.pdf).
20. Uganda AIDS Control Programme (ACP), *Medium-Term Plan for AIDS Control and Prevention* (WHO/Uganda Ministry of Health, 1986) 40.

21. WHO, *Guidelines for the Development of a National AIDS Prevention and Control Programme*, Series #1 (Geneva: WHO/AIDS, 1988).
22. WHO, *Guidelines*, 8.
23. GOU/ACP, *Medium-Term Plan*, 34.
24. Ibid., 34.
25. Ibid., 35.
26. GOU/Ministry of Health, *AIDS Surveillance Report* (Entebbe: Government Printers, June 1992) 2.
27. Dr Mwaka (Medical Officer for Health, Jinja District), personal interview, June 1992.
28. GOU/MOH/WHO, *Uganda ACP 1991 Plan and Budget* (Entebbe, 1991) 66.
29. GOU/MOH, *ACP Proposals for a Five-Year Action Plan 1987–1991* (Entebbe: Government Printers, 1987) 26.
30. GOU/MOH/WHO, 90.
31. Vali Jamal, 'Inequalities and Adjustment in Uganda', *Development and Change* 22.2 (1991): 325.
32. Tom Barton and Gimono Wamai, *Equity and Vulnerability: A Situation Analysis of Women, Adolescents and Children in Uganda* (Kampala: UNICEF, 1994) 101.
33. Dr J. Rhomushuna (Commisioner of Research for UAC), Personal Communication, Sept. 1992.
34. Uganda AIDS Commission Secretariat, *AIDS Control in Uganda: The Multisectoral Approach*, unpublished report (Kampala, 1993) 17.
35. Uganda AIDS Commission, *Multisectoral*, iv.
36. Centres for Disease Control, *HIV Prevention: Interventions and Evaluation*, unpublished report (USAID, 1992) 7.
37. Uganda ACP/MOH/GPA, *An Evaluation of Uganda ACPs IEC Activities*, unpublished draft report (Dec. 1991) 15.
38. Uganda ACP/MOH/GPA, *Evaluation*, 16.
39. Ibid., 25.
40. Personal interview, Walukuba, Jinja, June 1992.
41. Helen Epstein, 'AIDS: The Lesson of Uganda', *New York Review of Books* XLVIII.11 (5 July 2001): 18–19.
42. Epstein, 19.
43. Uganda AIDS Commission, *Multisectoral*.
44. Ibid., 10.
45. Ibid., 11.
46. The overall financial need for the period 1994–1998 was estimated by the UAC to be just under US$500 million. Of this amount, $241.3 million had been committed as of 1993, of which the WB pledged US$70.7 million. Other contributions came from USAID ($25 million), UNICEF ($10 million), UNDP ($15 million), UNFPA ($6.6 million), WHO ($1.1 Million), EEC ($13.2 million), WFP ($22 million), Italy ($4 million), UNESCO ($36 million), and the Government of Uganda ($37.5 million). All figures are in US dollars. Uganda AIDS Commission Secretariat, *Uganda National Operational Plan for HIV/AIDS/STD Prevention, Care and Support 1994–1998* (Kampala, 1993) 89.

47. Uganda AIDS Commission, *Uganda National*, x.
48. Ibid., 25.
49. Ibid., 25.
50. Ibid., 4.
51. Ibid., 6.
52. Ibid., 12–13.
53. Ibid., 35.
54. J. B. Mugaju, ed., *An Analytical Review of Uganda's Decade of Reforms 1986–1996* (Kampala: Fountain Press, 1996) 80.
55. Mugaju, 8.
56. Ibid., 89.
57. Uganda AIDS Commission, *Multisectoral*, 39.
58. Ibid., 68.
59. Uganda AIDS Commission Secretariat/UNAIDS, *Uganda National Strategic Framework for HIV/AIDS Activities in Uganda* 2000/1–2005/6 (11 Nov. 2000).
60. Uganda AIDS Commission, *Multisectoral*, 40.
61. Save the Children Fund, *Enumeration and Needs Assessment of Orphans in Uganda*, unpublished report prepared for the Department of Social Rehabilitation (Kampala: SCF/Makerere University, 1991).
62. J. Seeley *et al.*, 'Family Support for AIDS Patients in a Rural Population in Southwest Uganda: How Much a Myth?' unpublished paper, Medical Research Council (UK) Programme on AIDS in Uganda (Entebbe: MRC/UVRI, 1992).
63. Personal interview with a 50-year-old woman in Bunga, Kampala, Oct. 1992, and a 16-year-old female on the outskirts of Jinja, June 1992.
64. Anthony Klouda, 'Shifting Patterns in International Financing for AIDS Programs', *AIDS in the World*, eds Jonathan Mann *et al.* (Cambridge: Harvard University Press, 1992) 795.
65. Annemike Vink, 'Coping Strategies among AIDS-Affected People in Kisoro District, Southwest Uganda', unpublished report prepared for the St Frances Hospital (Mutolere: Kisoro, 1996) 35.
66. Vink, 41.
67. Ibid., 46.
68. Ibid., 45.
69. Ibid., 45.
70. Uganda AIDS Commision Secretariat, *The National Strategic Framework for HIV/AIDS Activities 1998–2002* (1998): 53.
71. Lee Rosner, personal interview, Kampala, Oct. 1992.
72. The New Vision, 'Uganda – Free HIV Drugs for All' (8 Aug. 2003), reproduced in *Medilinks Health News* (http://www.medilinks.org/news/news2.asp?page=3&NewsID=3512).
73. BBC News Online, 'AIDS Drugs Deal for Uganda' (3 Dec. 2000).
74. Uganda AIDS Commission, *Strategic Framework, 1998–2002*, 20–26.
75. AMREF-Uganda, *Inventory of Agencies with HIV/AIDS Interventions in Uganda 2001* (AMREF/UAC, July 2001) 29.
76. Extracted from notes on an interview with Dr Nelson Sewankambo, Oct. 1992.

Conclusion: AIDS, Human Rights, and Global Inequality

> Unlike women's work, the market economy is disconnected from daily physical realities; its operational imperatives bear no relation to people's needs; its exponential 'growth' trajectory even kills off its own future options.
>
> Ariel Salleh, *Ecofeminisim as Politics: Nature, Marx and the Postmodern*

Sub-Saharan Africa, despite over two decades of neoliberal economic and social reforms, has not seen a market-based recovery. As the latest collapsed round of WTO talks in Cancun, Mexico, illustrates, global economic reform has been a process rife with double standards. Rich countries have failed to deliver on their promises of opening up markets to developing countries and reducing agricultural protectionism, while largely ignoring the issue of the downward spiral of global commodity prices (accounting for three quarters of Africa's exports). They have focused on the enforcement of rich-country interests in intellectual property, particularly in the pharmaceutical sector, while 14 million people a year die of infectious diseases in developing countries. It is an understatement indeed that 'globalization has not yet worked for Africans'.

Instead of a market-based recovery, what many of the countries on the continent have seen instead is social, economic, and environmental collapse, while others have experienced escalating levels of violence and civil war, supported by the legacy of three decades of western-sponsored militarization. Social and economic crises have fuelled the emergence of new forms of masculinity, expressed in young boys

joining militaries and carrying sub-machine guns. Economic stagnation has underpinned 'ethnic' backlash, which has included the
'normalization' of sexual violence against and rape of women; a common feature of war in all places and at all times. Global economic
restructuring has served to reinforce and exacerbate existing gender,
class, and ethnic-based inequalities. At the level of ideology it valourizes
the qualities, behaviours, institutions, and practices associated with
men and masculinity – production for the market, competition, individual utility maximization – while devalourizing and/or disregarding
the 'female' realm of daily physical realities; of tending to the basic
needs for human survival and development. Neoliberalism has been
predicated on the exploitation of women's labour.

The re-casting of AIDS into a political economy perspective is
important for a number of reasons. First, it provides a challenge
to the mainstream approach to the epidemic in Africa and elsewhere
in the world, which has, as a defining feature, a neoliberal response to
the local impact of the epidemic; a tacit acceptance of the 'vicious
cycles of poverty' which is stated by Dr Sewankambo to be the main
impediment to the success of HIV/AIDS programmes. The institutional response has largely ignored the particular socio-economic
and political factors that have shaped the various epidemics within
the broader pandemic of AIDS – which in part explains the overwhelming emphasis on 'education for behaviour change'. Biomedical
experts initially set the global AIDS agenda, the main focus of which
has been on ever-more sophisticated cocktails to keep infection in
check for those who can afford them. Public health specialists were
brought in to design stopgap measures in the form of AIDS education
until the discovery of a vaccine or cure. All the while, life-saving
treatment has remained a luxury for the tiny minority who can pay
for it.

What does the Uganda case tell us? I have suggested that the unique
epidemiological pattern of HIV spread within Uganda's borders is
related to historical transformations in the economy and in social,
familial, and gender relations. British colonialism provided the slate
on which the script of the current epidemic could be written. The
historical transformations that underlie Uganda's current epidemic
were the evolution of a single-gender migrant labour economy; changes
in land tenure that rendered women more vulnerable combined with
increased demands on their labour created by the cash economy;

the breakdown of extended family systems; colonial health and social policies that did little to halt the spread of STIs but introduced a competing moral framework. In other countries of SSA, the script might be different, but in all cases historical legacies cannot be erased.

Post-independence developments provided the ideal environment in which, once introduced into human societies, HIV could flourish. The spatial and demographic pattern of HIV spread in Uganda was related to the growth of the 'magendo' economy and the different ways that men and women were drawn into it – men as long-distance traders and women as the service providers of these men. In war-torn areas such as Luwero and Gulu, the spread of HIV was hastened by escalating levels of sexual violence, lawlessness and social disruption. Once the virus took hold, its spread into the rural areas in the districts of highest HIV concentration had a certain inevitability, given the high level of movement between town and countryside, the long latency period of the virus in the body, continued high levels of STIs and compromised immunity, and the almost complete lack of basic health care services and disease surveillance at the time. The appearance of HIV in Uganda coincided with the end of 20 years of turmoil and mismanagement of the country, and the beginning of the country's reconstruction. The vacuum in development assistance was quickly filled by donor organizations, who, by virtue of a weak state, had a wide space in which to determine the shape of the institutional response.

In Uganda, the institutional response to the HIV/AIDS epidemic at the outset reflected the routine medical response of the WHO to the global pandemic. The response to HIV/AIDS began with wholly appropriate standardized medical interventions: setting up a surveillance system; cleaning up the blood supply; educating health workers on the main transmission routes and protocols for safe treatment; supplying clinics and hospitals with supplies such as needle-point sterilizers, protective gloves, and gowns. However appropriate, the constant difficulties encountered by the Uganda ACP to successfully implement even the most basic of policies, such as supplying protective gloves to health clinics, was a reflection of the structural weaknesses in service delivery. The problem, however, was not simply a matter of 'improving technical capacity'. The re-establishment of public health care was taking place in a context in which the cash-starved MOH was being told to trim expenditures and introduce user fees.

Government employees supplemented their salaries through growing their own food, engaging in petty trade, setting up private practice, and charging 'informal' fees for service.

The main focus on the side of prevention was on education, which, at the outset, was also appropriate, although the content of and approach to AIDS education was far from unproblematic. Sexual behaviour was understood to be static belief systems having no relation to the broader social, economic and political organization of Ugandan society. At the root of the behavioural change model of AIDS control and prevention was the understanding that what constituted 'normal' sexuality was monogamy within the confines of the nuclear family; overcoming or controlling sexual behaviour through IEC was the central focus of AIDS prevention in a society where there was little in the way of enabling social environment to support such changes. The widespread 'promiscuity' of Africans found its parallel in the gay communities of the West, where 'deviant' sexuality defined the research agendas of the mid-1980s.

At the level of AIDS expertise, breaking out of the 'health and education' focus of the dominant analytical approach has proven to be difficult. The approach of the ACP, however, did evolve from a strict focus on medical interventions and individual behaviour change to a more nuanced understanding of the socio-economic context of high-risk behaviour. Also reflected in the multisectoral strategy was a concern for the growing impact of the epidemic. Concerns that all sectors of society – agriculture, industry, health, education, the military – might be affected by AIDS morbidity and mortality, that the burgeoning number of AIDS orphans might create social instability and rising crime rates, and that women – the backbone of the subsistence economy and the main caregivers of the HIV infected – were particularly vulnerable resulted in a broadening of the definition and scope of AIDS interventions. All sectors were to become involved in AIDS prevention in Uganda – programmes were mainstreamed into all government departments, and the private sector was asked to take on greater responsibility. It was deemed that individual women needed to be 'empowered' through the establishment of income generation, made possible through better access to microcredit and training.

While the impact of HIV/AIDS morbidity and mortality throughout different sectors of society became a major focus of research, there was very little change in policies in Uganda and elsewhere to mitigate that impact. The spread and the consequences of HIV/AIDS have been largely understood as separate and distinct from broader macro-economic context which shapes the life chances of ordinary people in the cities and the countryside in profound ways. Responsibility for the local impact has fallen upon the shoulders of the affected communities themselves, as the Hope Clinic example so clearly demonstrates. The community response in many instances provides the basics – soap, school fees, home-care support, seeds, legal assistance – in a societal context in which the basics are considered private goods. NGOs and local grassroots organizations working in the districts have not been able to fill the vacuum created by the absence of the state in the provision of basic services and by the conditions of deep poverty that have remained relatively constant despite the infusions of development assistance, debt relief, state reform, and privatization. The 'local response' may be more relevant to the needs of hard-hit communities, but services are extremely unevenly distributed. The deeper the movement into the countryside, the poorer the social safety net provided by international development assistance and local charity. Circumscribing NGO and grassroots initiatives is the historical legacy of the bifurcated state, as well as the boundaries imposed by Uganda's Social Sector Strategy which have been part and parcel of IMF/WB restructuring.

There have been some successes during the last two decades of HIV/AIDS control in Uganda. There is a high level of awareness of HIV/AIDS. There is a strong political commitment and a govern-ment policy of openness to AIDS. Declining HIV prevalence rates have been observed among pregnant women attending antenatal clinics in some sentinel survey sites. There has been increased demand for voluntary testing facilities, and more couples are testing before marriage. Within the limitations circumscribed by the historical legacy of colonialism and the immediate post-colonial period, by a macroeconomic policy framework that places strict limitations on social sector expenditure, by a state which, despite a movement towards reform, remains the main avenue for individuals and social groups who aspire to political and economic domination, the past decade of AIDS control can be viewed as a success. Uganda is doing far better than its neighbours. Within the development community in Uganda, there is a level of debate that inspires optimism, and many committed and critical people are found at all levels.

This being said, it is still the case that the institutional response to AIDS in Uganda cannot address the broader factors that continue to put people at risk; nor does it come even close to mitigating the devastating impacts on the hardest-hit communities. The consequences of the epidemic will continue to be felt for years to come. AIDS articulates with other structural and social forces within communities in Uganda to create vicious circles. Declines in subsistence agricultural production result in deeper impoverishment and an increase in diseases associated with malnutrition. Declines in cash income combined with increased need for labour result in girls, before boys, being pulled from school, severely limiting their life chances and placing them at risk in the future. The movement of widows and orphans to urban areas in search of economic opportunities, where many will likely resort to 'high-risk behaviour' for sheer survival, adds further fuel to the epidemic. At a macrolevel, the declines in productive capacity mean that social expenditure, already woefully inadequate, will continue to be so.

The Ugandan case illustrates the limitations of an AIDS control strategy focused principally around education for behaviour change. Certain people are more able to act upon their knowledge than others. Single urban men who can afford condoms can choose to use them; they are less of an option for women whose social standing and self-worth is related to their ability to conceive a child; for married women whose husbands move to and from the village and who are raising their children in economically precarious circumstances; for women who suspect their husbands are infected but cannot say 'no' for fear of violence or abandonment; for others who simply cannot afford condoms. A recurring sentiment, expressed in interviews and in more casual conversation, was that AIDS was just another problem to face, and abstinence was difficult when sex is one of the few joys in life. 'Let me at least enjoy my life now, if I am to die soon of AIDS' were the words of one young shopkeeper in Kampala. For the invisible nurses – women in rural areas who are shouldering the main burden of the epidemic through their care of sick relatives and orphans – the response also has little to offer them. Certain interventions in the AIDS sector have begun to address the structural factors shaping the risk environment for AIDS, such as the law on violence against women and property rights, but the enforcement of laws is dependent on knowledge of the law and strong institutions to uphold them.

Although the Ugandan case offers more than simply vertical and technical solutions, the care of AIDS patients and the responsibility for mitigating the economic and social impact of AIDS deaths largely falls to 'the community'. The response reflects the neoliberal political agenda to the extent that an underlying assumption is that the role of the state is to enable, guide, and oversee, rather than to provide services. The great burden of coping with the epidemic falls on women who are 'empowered' to 'cope better' through community-based strategies. The radical discourse of PHC has been appropriated by the major institutions – but what 'empowerment' means is that 'communities' are essentially on their own. In the context of increased dependency ratios, AIDS-related productivity losses, shifting demographics and the privatization of health and other social services, prospects for the realization of the full potential of the economy through vigorous economic reform seem rather grim, caring for AIDS patients at home somewhat ill-conceived.

The ideological partner to the globalization of finance and production has been the undermining of collective responsibility for the social and economic well-being of societies, of the principles of universality, and of the exercise of basic human rights. In this context, the failures of the system are viewed as the sole responsibility of the individual, no longer the system or collectivity. AIDS can be considered a pandemic of globalization to the extent that its victims on a global scale increasingly are those who live on the margins, who have been displaced and excluded by processes originating from a politics of fragmentation which renders difficult any sort of collective vision for a just society: the urban poor living in unregulated settlements of Bombay and Sao Paulo without access to a living wage, proper housing, sanitation, and basic health services; women in Thailand, Nairobi, and Lyantonde who resort to transactional sex as one of the few strategies of survival open to them and their children; and poor black women in Harlem and Los Angeles who are members of the growing US underclass. New strategies and policies have emerged to address the human consequences of globalization – to attempt to impose stability in the face of increasing destabilization. The emerging discourse of the global AIDS pandemic as a crisis of 'national security' in the United States is reflected in their bypassing of the chronically cash-strapped Global AIDS and Health Fund in favour of its own bilateral programmes which will likely reflect the new focus of the Bush Administration on stricter monitoring of US-funded NGOs whose activities are inimical to US strategic interests and free-market principles. The American Enterprise Institute and the Federalist Society, right-wing think tanks with close ties to the Bush Administration, are launching NGO Watch, a website to reel in the power of NGOs that are not acting as an arm of US foreign policy. According to Health Global Access Project, there are suspicions that Bush's pledge of $15 billion over 5 years for HIV/AIDS in Africa and the Caribbean is little more than a slush fund for US-based pharmaceutical companies, and a vehicle to dictate abstinence in African and Caribbean communities.

In the meantime, the factors that fuel the spread of HIV are not considered proper targets for intervention. In essence, policies are designed to counter the destabilization caused by AIDS – biological, social, economic – to 'empower' the individual to better cope with his or her infection and imminent death, or to protect himself or herself from infection. The hegemonic understanding of African AIDS has failed to acknowledge that the vested interests that underlie the current global order contribute to the pattern and spread of HIV and disease, and the ability of communities to 'cope'.

The actual success of the global institutional response to AIDS in Africa, particularly to alleviate the impact of the epidemic in the hardest-hit communities, likely lies outside the AIDS-specific multi-sectoral strategies, but more firmly in the evolution of a just global order that sees the protection of the exercise of basic human rights not just as the responsibility of the individual nation-state. In our increasingly globalized world, it is the far-from-invisible hand of the market – the decisions of a particular epistemic community which views both patriarchy and capitalism as 'natural' – that shapes the local conditions which determine who has access to the exercise of basic human rights. Corporations, multilateral institutions, and IFIs are as culpable of human rights violations as African leaders and other individuals, yet come under little scrutiny. The growing global resistance to neoliberalism, in general, and to its brutal manifestations in African communities as reflected in the 'AIDS crisis' perhaps is reason for optimism. There is a greater awareness of the fact that global health and global trade are not distinct. The power of the civil society movement demanding access to treatment has resulted in intense pressure for reform within both the WTO and the individual nation-states. The debate itself has broadened and deepened; health is increasingly viewed as dependent on a broad range of needs and not just access to medicines, including control over one's production, adequate food, water and shelter, a secure physical environment, and bodily autonomy and integrity – the basic biological and developmental needs of all individuals. There is a growing awareness that the present practices and institutions of global system are not democratic, and that they are inimical to the protection of basic human rights – to truly sustainable growth and human development. But it is an optimism that is tempered by the fact that, ultimately, the AIDS epidemic will likely have come and gone before any genuine improvement has been made in the lives of the urban and rural poor in Uganda and elsewhere on the African continent.

Appendix

List of professionals in the HIV/AIDS sector interviewed in Uganda: June–December 1992

Mrs M. Owor, Coordinator, School Health Project ACEO.
Dr W. Naamara, Director, ACP, Ministry of Health.
Dr S. Kalibbala, STD Control Programme, Uganda Ministry of Health.
Dr Lwanga, Director, UAC.
Dr T. Barton, Technical Advisor, CHDC, Mulago Hospital.
Dr Mwaga, Head of Women's Studies, Makerere University.
Bonnie Keller, Planning Advisor, Ministry of Women and Development.
Marble Magezi, Public Relations Officer, TASO.
Donna Flanigan, IEC Advisor, GPA.
Dr N. Sewankambo, co-investigator, Lyantonde Project.
Dr J. Rwomushana, Research Coordinator, UAC.
Narathius Asinguirre, School of Social Work and Social Admin., Makerere University.
Janet Seeley, Medical Anthropologist, MRC/UVRI.
Daan Mulder, MRC/UVRI Researcher on Social Aspects of AIDS.
Donna Kabatesi, Acting Director, STD Control Unit, Mulago Hospital.
Jaques Homesy, Physician, MSF.
Carol Jaenson, SYFA, UNICEF.
Dr Adjai, Dept. of Statistics, Institute of Statistics and Applied Economics, Makerere University.
Lee Rosner, Project Manager, AIDS Prevention and Control Project, IEL.
Mr Tumushabe, Project Officer, AIDS Prevention and Control Project, IEL.
Harriet Burungi, Anthropogist, MISR.
Abbey Sebina-Nalwanga, social researcher on AIDS Projects, MISR.
Daniel Iga, Rakai Project, DANIDA.
Janet Nakuti, Researcher, Lyantonde Project.
Cheryl Walker, Director, CHIPS.
Joseph Lister, Project Officer, RAIN.
Joan Laroza, Health and Population Officer, USAID.
Hans Ehrenstrahle, Health Officer, World Bank.
Joyce Butera, Councillor, Rakai Project.
Godfrey Mukasa, Researcher, Lyantonde Project.
Dr J. T. M. Mwaka, District Medical Officer of Health, Jinja.
Mrs Tuma, RC4 Women's Representative, Jinja.
Robert Kelly, Project Officer, Rakai Project.

Mrs Katende, TASO Community Trainer.
Mary Mukajanka, Senior Nursing Officer, Mpummude Health Clinic.
Juliet Jogole, Counsellor, AIC, Jinja.
Naomi Afandula, Secretary, National Council of Women, Jinja District.

Bibliography

Adam, Christopher. 'Redesigning the Aid Contract: Donors' Use of Performance Indicators in Uganda.' *World Development* 30 (Dec. 2002): 2045–56.

Ahlberg, B. M. 'Is There a Distinct African Sexuality? A Critical Response to Caldwell.' *Africa.* 64.2 (1994): 220–36.

Ahluwalia, D. P. S. *Plantations and the Politics of Sugar in Uganda.* Kampala: Fountain Press, 1995.

Alagiri, Priya, Todd Summers, and Jennifer Kates. 'Global Spending on HIV/AIDS in Resource-Poor Settings.' The Henry J. Kaiser Family Foundation, July 2002.

AMREF-Uganda. *Inventory of Agencies with HIV/AIDS Interventions in Uganda 2001.* AMREF/UAC, July 2001.

Amuwo, Kunle. 'Globalization, NEPAD and the Governance Question in Africa.' *African Studies Quarterly Online Journal* (2002) (http://web.africa.ufl.edu/asq/v6/v6i3a4.htm).

Ankrah, Maxine. 'The Impact of AIDS on City/Town and Village Behavior in Uganda.' Conference paper, 5th Annual conference on AIDS. Montreal: June 1989.

——. 'AIDS and the Social Side of Health.' *Social Science and Medicine* 32.9 (1991): 967–80.

Appadurai, Arjun, ed. *Globalization.* Durham: Duke University Press, 2001.

Armstrong, Jill. 'Socioeconomic Implications of AIDS in Developing Countries.' *Finance and Development* (Dec. 1991): 14–17.

——. 'Uganda's AIDS Crisis: Its Implications for Development.' *World Bank Country Report.* Washington, DC: World Bank, 1994.

Attaran, Amir and Lee Gillespie White. 'Do Patents for Antiretroviral Drugs Constrain Access to Treatment in Africa.' *JAMA* 286 (17 Oct. 2001): 1186–92.

Baldo, Mariella, and Antonio Jorge Cabral. 'Low Intensity Wars and the Social Determination of HIV Transmission: The Search for a New Paradigm to Guide Research and Control of the HIV/AIDS Pandemic.' Eds Zena Stein and Anthony Zwi. *Action on AIDS in Southern Africa.* Maputo Conference on 'Health in Transition in Southern Africa' (Apr. 1990).

Barnett, Tony and Alan Whiteside. 'The Social and Economic Impact of HIV/AIDS in Poor Countries: A Review of Standards and Practices.' *Progress in Development Studies* 1.2 (2001): 151–70.

——. *AIDS in the Twenty-First Century: Disease and Globalization.* Basingstoke: Palgrave Macmillan, 2002.

Barnett, Tony and Piers Blaikie. *AIDS in Africa: Its Present and Future Impact.* London: Belhaven Press, 1992.

Barton, John H. 'Differentiated Pricing of Patented Products.' *WHO Commission on Macroeconomics and Health Working Paper Series* No. WG4: 2 (2001).

Barton, Tom and Gimono Wamai. *Equity and Vulnerability: A Situation Analysis of Women, Adolescents and Children in Uganda.* Kampala: UNICEF, 1994.

Basaza, Robert and Darlison Kaija. 'The Impact of HIV/AIDS on Children: Lights and Shadows in the "Successful Case" of Uganda.' Ed. Giovanni Andrea Cornia. *AIDS, Public Policy, and Child Well-Being.* UNICEF, June 2002.

Bassett, Mary and Marvellous Mhloyi. 'Women and AIDS in Zimbabwe: The Making of an Epidemic.' *International Journal of Health Service* 21.1 (1991): 143–56.

Bayart, Jean-Francois. *The State in Africa: The Politics of the Belly.* London: Longman, 1993.

Bayart, Jean-Francois, Stephen Ellis, and Beatrice Hibou. *The Criminalization of the State in Africa.* Oxford: James Currey, 1999.

Baylies, Carolyn. 'International Partnership in the Fight Against AIDS: Addressing Need and Redressing Injustice?' *Review of African Political Economy* 26.81 (1999): 387–94.

——. 'Overview: AIDS in Africa.' *Review of African Political Economy* 28.86 (2000): 487–500.

——. 'HIV/AIDS and Older Women in Zambia: Concern Over Self, Worry Over Daughters, Towers of Strength.' *Third World Quarterly* 23.2 (2002): 351–76.

Baylies, Carolyn and Janet Burja. 'Editorial: Special Issue on AIDS.' *Review of African Political Economy* 28.86 (2000): 483–86.

Benatar, Solomon. 'South Africa's Transition in a Globalizing World: HIV/AIDS as a Window and a Mirror.' *International Affairs* 77.2 (2001): 347–75.

Benatar, Solomon, Abdallah S. Daar, and Peter Singer. 'Global Health Ethics: A Rationale for Mutual Caring.' *International Affairs* 79.1 (2003): 107–38.

Beneria, Lourdes *et al.* 'Introduction: Globalization and Gender.' *Feminist Economics* 6. 3 (Nov. 2000): vii–xviii.

Bergeron, Suzanne. 'Political Economy Discourses of Globalization and Feminist Politics.' *Signs* 26 (2001): 983–1006.

Bettley, F. R. 'Venereal Disease Control in the East Africa Command.' *Journal of the Royal Army Medical Corps* 85.3 (1945): 109–16.

Bollinger, Lori, John Stover, and Vastha Kibirige. 'The Economic Impact of AIDS in Uganda.' Unpublished paper. The Futures Group International, Sept. 1999.

Bombelles, Tom. 'Facts and Figures on Patenting and Access in Africa.' Conference paper. American Society of Law, Medicine and Ethics Conference, 2001.

Bond, George C. *et al.*, eds. *AIDS in Africa and the Caribbean.* Boulder: Westview Press, 1997.

Boseley, Sarah. 'UN AIDS Fund Empty as US Offers $15bn.' *The Guardian Weekly* 6–12 Feb. 2003: 5.

Brittain, Victoria. 'A Nation that Hates its Women.' *New Statesman.* 24 June 2002.

Brown, Judith E., Okako B. Ayowa, and Richard C. Brown. 'Dry and Tight: Sexual Practices and Potential AIDS Risk in Zaire.' *Social Science and Medicine* 37.8 (1993): 989–94.

Buse, Kent and Gill Walt. 'Globalization and Multilateral Public–Private Health Partnerships: Issues for Health Policy.' Eds Kelly Lee, Kent Buse, and Suzanne Fustukian. *Health Policy in a Globalizing World*. Cambridge: Cambridge University Press, 2002.

Bush, Ray and Giles Mohan. 'Africa's Future: That Sinking Feeling.' *Review of African Political Economy* 28.88 (2001): 149–53.

Caldwell, John, Pat Caldwell, and Pat Quiggen. 'The Social Context of AIDS in Sub-Saharan Africa.' *Population and Development Review* 15.2 (1989): 185–234.

Campbell, Bonnie. 'Governance, Institutional Reform & the State: International Financial Institutions & Political Transition in Africa.' *Review of African Political Economy* 28.88 (2001): 155–76.

Centres for Disease Control. 'HIV Prevention: Interventions and Evaluation.' Unpublished report. USAID, 1992.

Chabal, Patrick and Jean-Pascal Daloz. *Africa Works: Disorder as Political Instrument*. Oxford: James Currey, 1999.

Chanock, Martin. 'Making Customary Law: Men, Women and Courts in Colonial Northern Rhodesia.' Eds Margaret Jean Hay and Marcia Wright. *African Women and the Law: Historical Perspectives*. Boston: Boston University Papers in Africa VII, 1982.

Chapman, Audrey R. 'The Human Rights Implications of Intellectual Property Protection.' *Journal of International Economic Law* (2002): 861–82.

Check, Erika. 'AIDS Vaccines: Back to Plan A.' *Nature* 423 (2003): 912–94.

Cheru, Fantu. 'Debt, Adjustment and the Politics of Effective Response to HIV/AIDS in Africa.' *Third World Quarterly* 23.2 (2002): 299–312.

Clark, Carolyn. 'Land and Food, Women and Power in Nineteenth Century Kikuyu.' *Africa* 50.4 (1980): 359–69.

Cohen, Jon. 'Deep Denial.' *The Sciences* 4.1 (Jan./ Feb. 2001): 20–24.

Comaroff, Jean. 'The Diseased Heart of Africa: Medicine, Colonialism and the Black Body.' Eds Shirley Lindenbaum and Margaret Lock. *Knowledge Power and Practice: The Anthropology of Medicine in Everyday Life*. Berkeley: University of California Press, 1993.

Cooke, Alexander. 'The Treatment of Ante-natal Syphilis in Kenya.' *East Africa Medical Journal* 6.1 (1929).

——. 'The Influence of Obstetrical Conditions on Vital Statistics in Uganda.' *East Africa Medical Journal* 9.11 (1933): 316–30.

Cornia, Giovanni A. 'Adjustment Policies 1980–85: Effects on Child Welfare.' Eds Cornia, Jolly and Stewart. *Adjustment with a Human Face, Volume 1*. Oxford: Clarendon Press, 1987.

Correa, Carlos M. 'Implementing National Public Health Policies in the Framework of WTO Agreements.' *Journal of World Trade* 34.5 (2000): 89–121.

Craig, John. 'Evaluating Privitisation in Zambia: A Tale of Two Processes.' *Review of African Political Economy* 27.85 (2000): 357–66.

Creese, Andrew. 'Cost-effectiveness of HIV/AIDS Interventions in Africa: A Systematic Review of the Evidence.' *The Lancet* 359 (11 May 2002): 1635–42.

Cullet, Philippe. 'Patents and Medicines: The Relationship between TRIPS and the Human Right to Health.' *International Affairs* 79.1 (2003): 139–60.

Dak, O. 'A Geographical Analysis of the Distribution of Migrants in Uganda.' Occasional Paper No. 11. Kampala: Department of Geography, Makerere University, 1968.

Dodge, Cole P. 'Health Implications of War in Uganda and Sudan.' *Social Science and Medicine* 31.6 (1990): 691–98.

Dodge, Cole P. and Magne Raundalen, eds. *War, Violence and Children in Uganda.* Oslo: Norwegian University Press, 1987.

Doyal, Lesley. *The Political Economy of Health.* London: Pluto Press, 1979.

——. 'Putting Gender into Health and Globalization Debates: New Perspectives and Old Challenges.' *Third World Quarterly* 23.2 (2002): 223–50.

du Guerny, J. 'AIDS and Agriculture in Africa: Can Agricultural Policy Make a Difference?' *Food, Nutrition and Agriculture* 25 (1999): 12–17 (ftp://ftp.fao.org/docrep/fao/X4390t/4390t03.pdf).

Dunlop, D. and S. Scheyer. 'Health Services and Development in Uganda.' Eds Paul Cole and Paul Wiebe. *Crisis in Uganda: The Breakdown of Health Services.* Oxford: Pergamon, 1985.

Elkan, Walter. *Migrants and Proletarians: Urban Labour in the Economic Development of Uganda.* London: Oxford University Press, 1960.

——. *The Economic Development of Uganda.* London: Oxford University Press, 1961.

Elson, Diane. 'The Impact of Structural Adjustment on Women: Concepts and Issues.' Report of the WID Programme of the Commonwealth Secretariat. May 1987.

Epstein, Helen. 'AIDS: The Lesson of Uganda.' *New York Review of Books* XLVIII.11 (15 July 2001): 18–23.

Epstein, Steven. *Impure Science: AIDS, Activism and the Politics of Knowledge.* Berkeley: University of California Press, 1996.

Escobar, Arturo. *Encountering Development: The Making and Unmaking of the Third World.* New Jersey: Princeton University Press, 1995.

Etienne, Mona. 'Women and Men, Cloth and Colonization: The Transformation of Production–Distribution Relations among the Baule.' Eds Mona Etienne and Eleanor Leacock. *Women and Colonization: Anthropological Perspectices.* New York: Praeger, 1980. 214–38.

Etienne, Mona and Eleanor Leacock, eds. *Women and Colonization: Anthropological Perspectices.* New York: Praeger, 1980.

Evans, Tony. 'A Human Right to Health?' *Third World Quarterly* 23.2 (2002): 197–215.

FAO. 'Food Supply Situation and Crop Prospects in Sub-Saharan Africa.' No. 3. Dec. 2002 (http://www.fao.org/giews/).

Farmer, Paul. *Infections and Inequalities: The Modern Plagues.* Berkeley: University of California Press, 2001.

——. *Pathologies of Power: Health, Human Rights, and the New War on the Poor.* Berkeley: University of California Press, 2003.

Feldman, Douglas. 'Editorial.' *Social Science and Medicine* 33.7 (1991): 783–85.

Ferguson, James. *The Anti-Politics Machine.* Minneapolis: University of Minnesota Press, 1994.

Forsythe, Steven, ed. *State of the Art: AIDS and Economics.* International AIDS Economics Network. July 2002.

Frommel, D. 'Editorial.' *Le Monde Diplomatique English Supplement to the Guardian* Jan. 2001: 11.

Furley, Oliver. 'Education in Post-independence Uganda: Change Amidst Strife.' Eds H. B. Hansen and M. Twaddle. *Uganda Now: Between Decay and Development.* London: James Currey, 1988.

Garrett, Laurie. *Betrayal of Trust.* New York: Hyperion, 2000.

Gill, Stephen. 'Globalization, Market Civilization and Disciplinary Neoliberalism.' *Millennium: Journal of International Studies* 24.3 (1995): 399–423.

Gill, Stephen, ed. *Gramsci, Historical Materialism and International Relations.* Cambridge: Cambridge University Press, 1993.

Global HIV Prevention Working Group. *Access to Prevention: Closing the Gap.* May 2003.

Godlee, Fiona. 'WHO in Retreat: Is It Losing Its Influence?' *British Medical Journal* 309. 6967 (1994): 1491–95.

——. 'WHO's Special Programmes: Undermining from above.' *British Medical Journal* 310.6973 (1995): 178–82.

——. 'WHO Reform and Global Health.' *British Medical Journal* 314.7091 (1997): 1359–60.

Gombay, Christopher. 'Canadian Non-governmental Organizations and CIDA: Whither Canadian NGOs?' Paper prepared for the Canadian Council on Social Development. 2002.

——. 'Eating Cities: The Politics of Everyday Life in Kampala, Uganda.' PhD thesis, University of Toronto, 1997.

Gordenker, Leon *et al.* 'International Cooperation and AIDS: A Report on Research Findings.' Conference paper. Annual Meetings of the International Study Association. Washington, 1994.

GOU. *Background to the Budget 1995/1996.* Entebbe: Government Printers, 1995.

GOU. *Final Results of the 1991 Population and Housing Census.* Entebbe: Government Printers, 1992.

GOU. *The Resistance Councils and Committees Statute 1987.* Entebbe: Government Printers, 1987.

GOU Ministry of Finance. *Background to the Budget 1991–1992.* Entebbe: Government Printers, 1991.

——. *The Way Forward I: Macroeconomic Strategy 1990–1995 and The Way Forward II: Medium Term Sectoral Strategy 1991–1995.* Entebbe: Government Printers, 1992.

GOU Ministry of Health. *ACP Proposal for a Five-year Action Plan 1987–1991.* Entebbe: Government Printers, 1987.

——. *AIDS Surveillance Report June 1992.* Entebbe: Government Printers, 1992.

——. 'Uganda STD Control Project: A Proposal to the World Bank.' Unpublished. Oct. 1993.

GOU Ministry of Health/WHO. *Uganda ACP 1991 Plan and Budget.* Entebbe: Health Education Printing Unit, 1991.

Gray, Andy and Jenni Smit. 'Improving Access to HIV-related Drugs in South Africa: A Case of Colliding Interests.' *Review of African Political Economy* 28.86 (Dec. 2000): 583–90.

Green, Reginald. 'Magendo in the Political Economy of Uganda: Pathology, Parallel System or Dominant Sub-mode of Production?' Discussion paper 165. Institute of Development Studies, University of Sussex, 1981.

Greenhill, Romilly. 'New World Bank Reports Confirm that HIPC Initiative is Failing.' *Jubilee Research*. 29 Apr. 2002.

Gruskin, Sofia and Daniel Tarantola. *Health and Human Rights*. Francois-Xavier Bagnoud Center Working Paper No. 10. Boston: FXB Center, 2000 (http://www.hsph.harvard.edu/fxbcenter/FXBC_WP--Gruskin_and_Tarantola.pdf).

Guyer, Jane. 'Female Farming and the Evolution of Food Production Patterns amongst the Beti of South Central Cameroon.' *Africa* 50.4 (1980): 341–55.

Hafkin, Nancy J. and Edna Bay. *Women in Africa: Studies in Social and Economic Change*. Stanford: Stanford University Press, 1976.

Hansen, H. B. and M. Twaddle, eds. *Uganda Now: Between Decay and Development*. London: James Currey, 1988.

——. *Changing Uganda: The Dilemmas of Structural Adjustment and Revolutionary Change*. London: James Currey, 1991.

Harrington, Mark. 'Brazil: What Went Right? The Global Access to Treatment and the Issue of Compulsory Licensing.' Conference paper. 10th National Meeting of People Living with HIV and AIDS. Rio de Janiero, Brazil: 3 Nov. 2000.

Harrod, Jeffrey. 'United Nations Specialized Agencies: From Functionalist Intervention to International Cooperation?' Eds J. Harrod and N. Schrijver. *The UN Under Attack*. New York: Gower Press, 1991.

Hay, Margaret Jean and Marcia Wright, eds. *African Women and the Law: Historical Perspectives*. Boston: Boston University Papers on Africa VII, 1982.

Hearn, Julie. 'The NGO-ization of Kenyan Society: USAID and the Restructuring of Health Care.' *Review of African Political Economy* 25.75 (1998): 89–101.

Held, David and Anthony McGrew, eds. *The Global Transformations Reader*. Malden: Blackwell Publishers, 2000.

Helleiner, Gerry. 'Marginalization and/or Participation: Africa in Today's Global Economy.' *Canadian Journal of African Studies* 36.3 (2002): 531–50.

Heywood, Mark. 'Drug Access, Patents and Global Health: "Chaffed and Waxed Sufficient."' *Third World Quarterly* 23.2 (2002): 217–31.

Hogle, Janice, ed. 'What Happened in Uganda? Declining Prevalence, Behavior Change, and the National Response.' USAID Project Lessons Learned Case-Study. Sept. 2002.

Hulme, David and Michael Edwards, eds. *NGOs, States and Donors: Too Close for Comfort?* New York: St Martin's Press, 1997.

Human Rights Watch. *The War Within the War: Sexual Violence Against Women and Girls in Eastern Congo*. New York, 2002.

——. 'Double Standards: Women's Property Rights Violations in Kenya.' *Human Rights Watch Report* 15.5(A) (Aug. 2003).

——. 'Just Die Quietly: Domestic Violence and Women's Vulnerability to HIV in Uganda.' *Human Rights Watch Report* 15.15(A) (Aug. 2003).

Hunt, Charles. 'Social vs. Biological: Theories on Transmission of AIDS in Africa.' *Social Science and Medicine* 42.9 (1996): 1283–96.

Hunter, Susan. 'Orphans as a Window on the AIDS Epidemic in Sub-Saharan Africa: Initial Results and Implications from a Study of Uganda.' *Social Science and Medicine* 31.6 (1990): 681–90.

Ibhawoh, Bonny. 'Structural Adjustment, Authoritarianism, and Human Rights in Africa.' *Comparative Studies of South Asia, Africa and the Middle East* XIX.1 (1999): 158–67.

International Crisis Group. *HIV/AIDS as a Security Issue*. Washington/Brussels: ICG, 19 June 2001 (http://www.intl-crisis-group.org/projects/issues/hiv-aids/reports/A400321-19062001.pdf).

International Labour Organization. 'AIDS a Major Threat to the World of Work.' 8 June 2000 (http://www.ilo.org/public/english/protetion/trav/aids/index.htm).

Jacobson, Harold K. 'WHO: Medicine, Regionalism and Managed Politics.' Eds Robert Cox and Harold K. Jacobson. *The Anatomy of Influence: Decision Making in International Organizations*. New Haven: Yale University Press, 1973. 175–215.

Jamal, Vali. 'Inequalities and Adjustment in Uganda.' *Development and Change* 22.2 (1991): 321–37.

Janjua, Harinder. *The Best Chance We Have: The Global Fund to Fight AIDS, TB and Malaria*. Action Aid, 16 June 2003.

Joint Evaluation Team. 'The Report of the Joint Evaluation of the Uganda AIDS Commission and Secretariat.' Unpublished. Kampala, 1992.

Joint Session of the EXEC Boards of UNDP/UNFPA, UNICEF and WFP. 'HIV/AIDS: Addressing the Recommendations of the UNAIDS Five Year Evaluation.' 9 June 2003.

Kalule, Josephine *et al.* 'A Report of the AIDS Information Centre Symposium.' Uganda Management Institute. 16 Mar. 1995.

Kanbur, Ravi. 'Aid, Conditionality and Debt in Africa.' Ed. Finn Tarp. *Foreign Aid and Development: Lessons Learned and Directions for the Future*. London: Routledge, 2000.

Kanyeihamba, George. 'Power that Rode Naked in Uganda Under the Muzzle of a Gun.' Eds H. B. Hansen and M. Twaddle. *Uganda Now: Between Decay and Development*. London: James Currey, 1988.

Kendegeya-Kayondo, J. F., S. D. K. Sempala and J. Whitworth. 'Medical Research Council (UK), ODA (UK) Uganda Virus Research Institute Programme Annual Report for 1995.' Entebbe: Apr. 1996.

Khadiagala, Gilbert M. 'State Collapse and Reconstruction in Uganda.' Ed. William Zartman. *Collapsed States: The Disintegration and Restoration of Legitimate Authority*. London: Lynne Rienner, 1995.

Kiirya, Stephen. 'HIV/AIDS in Uganda: A Comprehensive Analysis of the Epidemic and the Response.' Uganda AIDS Commission, 1998.

Killewo, J. T. Z. *et al. Behavioral and Epidemiological Aspects of AIDS Research in Tanzania*. Workshop proceedings. Dar es Salaam: 6–8 Dec. 1989.

Klein, Naomi. 'Reclaiming the Commons.' *New Left Review* 9 (2001).

Klouda, Anthony. 'Shifting Patterns in International Financing for AIDS Programs.' Eds Jonathan Mann *et al. AIDS in the World*. Cambridge: Harvard University Press, 1992. 787–801.

——. 'Organizations and AIDS: The Development of Coping Responses.' Conference paper. Meeting of the African Studies Association. Toronto, 4 Nov. 1994.

Konde-Lule, Joseph, M. Musagara, and S. Musgrave. 'Focus Group Interviews About AIDS in Rakai District of Uganda.' *Social Science and Medicine* 37.5 (1993): 679–84.

Krieger, Nancy. 'Epidemiology and the Web of Causation: Has Anyone Seen the Spider?' *Social Science and Medicine* 39 (1994): 887–903.

Kumaranayake, L. *et al.* 'Preliminary Estimates of the Cost of Expanding TB, Malaria and HIV/AIDS Activities for Sub-Saharan Africa.' *WHO Commission on Macroeconomics and Health Working Paper Series* WG5: 26 (2001).

Labov, Teresa G. 'NGOs, HIV/AIDS Control and Reproductive Health in East Africa.' *The International Journal of Sociology and Social Policy* 22.4–6 (2002): 100–133.

Lateef, K. Sawar. 'Structural Adjustment in Uganda: The Initial Experience.' Eds H. B. Hansen and M. Twaddle. *Changing Uganda*. London: James Currey, 1993.

Laurell, A. C. and Olivia Lopez Arellano. 'Market Commodities and Poor Relief: The World Bank Proposal for Health.' *International Journal of Health Services* 26.1 (1996): 1–18.

Lawrence, Peter, ed. *World Recession and the Food Crisis in Africa*. London: James Currey, 1986.

Lee, Kelley and Hilary Goodman. 'Global Policy Networks: The Propagation of Health Care Financing Reform Since the 1980s.' Eds Kelley Lee, Kent Buse, and Suzanne Fustukian. *Health Policy in a Globalizing World*. Cambridge: Cambridge University Press, 2002: 97–119.

Lee, Kelley, Kent Buse, and Suzanne Fustukian, eds. *Health Policy in a Globalizing World*. Cambridge: Cambridge University Press, 2002.

Lewicky, Nan and Maggie Wheeler. 'HIV/AIDS and Adolescents: Key Findings from the Youth HIV/AIDS Baseline Survey of Seven Districts of Uganda.' Kampala: USAID, July 1996.

Lewis, Stephen. 'AIDS, Conflict, Poverty: The Challenge for Canada and the UN.' *Canadian Development Report* (2000): 2–9.

Love, James with Michael Palmedo. 'Sub-Saharan African Patents by Population and Income: Draft.' Consumer Project on Technology. 6 Oct. 2001.

Madraa, Elizabeth and Major Ruranga-Rubaramira. 'HIV Prevention Works: The Uganda Case-Study.' Conference paper. 11th International Conference on AIDS. Vancouver, 7–12 July 1996.

Malamba, S. *et al.* 'Risk Factors for HIV-1 Infection in Adults in a Rural Ugandan Community: A Case-control Study.' *AIDS* 8.2 (1994).

Mamdani, Mahmood. *Politics and Class Formation in Uganda*. London: Monthly Review Press, 1976.

——. 'Uganda: Contradiction of the IMF Programme and Perspective.' *Development and Change* 22 (1991): 427–67.

——. *Citizen and Subject: Contemporary Africa and the Legacy of Late Colonialism*. New Jersey: Princeton University Press, 1996.

Mandala, Elias. 'Peasant Cotton Agriculture, Gender and Inter-generational Relationships: The Lower Tchiri Valley of Malawi, 1906–1940.' *African Studies Review* 25.2–3 (1982): 27–43.

Manji, Ambreena. 'Capital, Labour and Land Relations in Africa: A Gender Analysis of the World Bank's Policy Research Report on Land Institutions and Land Policy.' *Third World Quarterly* 24.1 (2003): 97–114.

Manji, Firoze and Carl O'Coill. 'The Missionary Position: NGOs and Development in Africa.' *International Affairs* 78.3 (2002): 567–83.

Mann, Jonathan and Kathleen Kay. 'Confronting the Pandemic: The WHO's Global Programme on AIDS, 1986–1989.' *AIDS* 5 (1991): s221–s229.

Mann, Jonathan, Daniel Tarantola, and Thomas Netter, eds. *AIDS in the World*. Cambridge: Harvard University Press, 1992.

Marchand, Marianne H. and Anne Sisson Runyan, eds. *Gender and Global Restructuring: Sightings, Sites and Resistances*. London: Routledge, 2000.

Marseille, Elliot, Paul Hofmann, and James Kahn. 'HIV Prevention before HAART in Sub-Saharan Africa.' *The Lancet* 359.9320 (2002): 1851–56.

Mbilinyi, Marjorie. 'City and Countryside in Colonial Tanganyika.' *Economic and Political Weekly* XX.43 (1985): 88–96.

McCrombie, Susan. 'Results from a Second Survey of AIDS-Related Knowledge, Attitudes and Practices Among Workers in Uganda.' Unpublished report. AIDSCOM, 1991.

McCrombie, Susan and Robert Hornik. 'Evaluation of a Workplace-based Peer Education Program Designed to Prevent AIDS in Uganda.' Unpublished report. AIDSCOM in collaboration with the Federation of Uganda Employers and Experiment in International Living, Apr. 1992.

McGrath, J. *et al*. 'Anthropology and AIDS: The Cultural Context of Sexual Risk Behaviour among Urban Women in Kampala, Uganda.' *Social Science and Medicine* 36.4 (1993): 429–39.

Médecins Sans Frontières. 'Patents do Matter in Africa According to NGOs: Joint statement by Oxfam, Treatment Action Campaign, Consumer Project on Technology (CPT), Médecins Sans Frontières (MSF) and Health GAP.' Press release. MSF, 17 Oct. 2001 (http://www.accessmed-msf.org/prod/publications.asp?scntid=171020011428553&contenttype=PARA&).

Médecins Sans Frontières Campaign for Access to Essential Medicines. 'AIDS Treatment Scale-Up Efforts Threatened: Donor Countries Fail to Fill the Funding Gap.' 16 July 2003 (http://www.accessmed-msf.org/prod/publications.asp?scntid=16720031828312&contenttype=PARA&).

Meinert, Lotte, Imelda Tamwesigire, and Proscovia Musumba. 'An Evaluation Report on SYFA Straight Talk Mass Media Effort.' Unpublished report. Kampala: Apr. 1995.

Mengisteab, Kidane and Ikubolajeh Logan, eds. *Beyond Economic Liberalization in Africa: Structural Adjustment and the Alternatives*. London: Zed Books, 1995.

Microcredit Summit Campaign. 'African Microenterprise AIDS Initiative.' (http://www.microcreditsummit.org/press/Africanmicro.htm).

Microcredit Summit Campaign. 'Microcredit Helps Ease the Burden of AIDS in Africa.' (http://www.microcreditsummit.org/press/AIDS.htm).

Mohan, Giles and Kristian Stokke. 'Participatory Development and Empowerment: The Dangers of Localism.' *Third World Quarterly* 21.2 (2000): 247–68.

Mohanty, Chandra Talpade, Ann Russo, and Lourdes Torres, eds. *Third World Women and the Politics of Feminism*. Bloomington: Indiana University Press, 1991.

Molnos, Angela, ed. *Cultural Source Materials for Population Planning in East Africa*. Vol. 2. Nairobi: East African Publishing House, 1972.

Mooney, Pat Roy. 'The Parts of Life: Agricultural Biodiversity, Indigenous Knowledge, and the Role of the Third System.' *Development Dialogue* Special Issue 1–2 (1996): 1–183.

Moore, David. 'Levelling the Playing Fields and Embedding Illusions: "Post-Conflict" Discourse and Neo-liberal "Development" in War-torn Africa.' *Review of African Political Economy* 27.83 (2000): 11–28.

Moser, Caroline and Fiona Clarke, eds. *Victims, Perpetrators or Actors? Gender, Armed Conflict and Political Violence*. London: Zed Books 2001.

Mugaju, J. B., ed. *An Analytical Review of Uganda's Decade of Reforms 1986–1996*. Kampala: Fountain Press, 1996.

Mukasa, G. *et al.* 'Who is Talking . . . Who is Listening? A Gender Analysis of Communications About AIDS and Sexuality in Rural Uganda.' Conference paper. 7th International Conference on AIDS in Africa. Yaounde: 8–11 Dec. 1992.

Mukwaya, A. B., *Land Tenure in Buganda: Present Day Tendencies*. Kampala: Eagle Press, 1953.

Mulder, Daan *et al.* 'HIV-1 Incidence and HIV-1 Associated Mortality in a Rural Ugandan Population Cohort.' *AIDS* 8 (1992): 87–92.

Munishi, Gaspar Kilala. 'Intervening to Address Constraints Through Health Sector Reforms in Tanzania: Some Gains and the Unfinished Business.' *Journal of International Development* 15 (2003): 115–31.

Muntemba, Maud. 'Women and Agricultural Change in the Railway Region of Zambia: Dispossession and Counterstrategies, 1930–1970.' Ed. Edna Bay. *Women and Work in Africa*. Boulder: Westview Press, 1982. 83–106.

Museveni, Yoweri. *What is Africa's Problem?* Kampala: NRM Publications, 1992.

Musisi, Nakanyike. 'Women, Elite Polygyny and Buganda State Formation.' *Signs* 16 (1991): 757–86.

Mutagamba, B. *et al.* 'Laying the Foundation for Core Change in High Risk Communities: Ethnography of a Lorry Stop in SW Uganda.' Conference paper. 7th International Conference on AIDS in Africa. Yaounde: 8–11 Dec. 1992.

Mutibwa, Phares. *Uganda Since Independence*. Kampala: Fountain Publishers, 1992.

Nabudere, Dani Wadada. 'External and Internal Factors in Uganda's Continuing Crisis.' Eds H. B. Hansen and M. Twaddle. *Uganda Now: Between Decay and Development*. London: James Currey, 1988.

Nagendo, Florence and Tom Barton. 'KAP Related to AIDS among Secondary Students in Kabarole District: A Qualitative Secondary Analysis.' Unpublished paper. Kampala: GTZ, 1992.

Nakuti, J. *et al.* 'If We Fear AIDS What Will We Eat? Women's Struggle for Economic Independence in a Rural Uganda Lorry Stop.' Conference paper. 7th International Conference on AIDS in Africa. Yaounde: 8–11 Dec. 1992.

Naples, Nancy and Manisha Desai, eds. *Women's Activism and Globalization*. New York: Routledge, 2002.

National Institutes of Health Office of AIDS Research. *Global AIDS Research Initiative and Strategic Plan*. Dec. 2000.

Nderitu, Terry. 'Balancing Pills and Patents: Intellectual Property and the HIV/AIDS Crisis.' *E-Law – Murdoch U Electronic Journal of Law* 8.3 (2001): 1–9 (http://www.murdoch.edu.au/elaw/issues/v8n3/nderitu83.html).

Ndikumana, Léonce. 'Beyond Good Intentions: Is U.S. Newly found Interest in Africa Real?' *Econ-Atrocity Bulletin* (2 Jan. 2003) (http://www.fguide.org/Bulletin/africa.htm).

Nnko, Soori *et al*. 'Tazania AIDS Care – Learning from Experience.' *Review of African Political Economy* 28.86 (2000): 547–57.

Nsutebu, Emmanuel Fru *et al*. 'Scaling-up HIV/AIDS and TB Home-based Care: Lessons from Zambia.' *Health Policy and Planning* 16.3 (2001): 240–47.

Nunn, Andrew J. *et al*. 'Risk Factors for HIV-1 Infection in Adults in a Rural Ugandan Community: A Population Study.' *AIDS* 8.1 (1994).

Obbo, Christine. 'Dominant Male Ideology and Female Options: Three East African Case-studies.' *Africa* 46.4 (1976): 371–88.

——. 'Stratification and the Lives of Women in Uganda.' Eds Claire Robertson and Iris Berger. *Women and Class in Africa*. New York: Holmes and Meier, 1986.

——. 'What Went Wrong in Uganda?' Eds H. B. Hansen and M. Twaddle. *Uganda Now*. London: James Currey, 1998.

Ochieng, E. O. 'Economic Adjustment Programs in Uganda 1985–89.' Eds H. B. Hansen and M. Twaddle. *Changing Uganda: The Dilemmas of Structural Adjustment and Revolutionary Change*. London: James Currey, 1991. 43–60.

Ohanyan, Anna. 'The Politics of Microcredit.' Case Study for the UN Vision Project on Global Public Policy Networks, 2000.

Okeyo, Achola Pala. 'Daughters of the Lakes and Rivers: Colonization and the Land Rights of Luo Women.' Eds Mona Etienne and Eleanor Leacock. *Women and Colonization: Anthropological Perspectives*. New York: Praeger, 1980.

Olowo Freers, Bernadette. 'Sexual Behavior Practices: Cultural and Social Aspects of Transmission of AIDS in Uganda.' Unpublished discussion paper, 1991.

Olowo-Freers, Bernadette and Thomas Barton. 'In Pursuit of Fulfillment: Studies of Cultural Diversity and Sexual Behavior in Uganda: An Overview Essay and Annotated Bibliography.' Unpublished report. Kampala: 1992.

O'Malley, Jeff. 'AIDS Service Organizations in Transition.' Eds Jonathon Mann *et al*. *AIDS in the World*. Cambridge: Harvard University Press, 1992. 774–87.

O'Manique, Colleen. 'Traditional Therapies and Biomedicine in Uganda.' *International Health Exchange Project Reports* 3 (Ottawa: 1989). 71–84.

——. 'Agriculture, Women and Structural Adjustment in Sub-Saharan Africa.' Unpublished paper. Toronto: June 1990.

——. 'Socio-economic and Gender Analysis: Jinja Municipality.' Unpublished report prepared for Jinja Municipality, Uganda, JVN Associates, 1994.

——. 'Liberalizing AIDS in Africa: The World Bank Role.' *Southern Africa Report* 11.4 (1996).

——. 'The Pandemic of Globalization', PhD thesis York University, Nov. 1997.

——. 'Engendering Health and Globalization: Neoliberalism and AIDS Crisis in Sub-Saharan Africa.' Conference paper. Annual Meeting of the International Studies Association. Portland: Feb. 2003.

——. 'Global Neoliberalism and AIDS Policy: International Responses to Africa's Pandemic.' Forthcoming in *Studies in Political Economy* (Jan. 2004).

O'Manique, John. *The Origins of Justice: The Evolution of Morality, Human Rights and Law*. Philadelphia: University of Pennsylvania Press, 2003.

Onimode, Bade, ed. *The IMF, the World Bank and African Debt: The Social and Political Impact*. London: Zed Books, 1989.

Oppenheimer, Gerald. 'In the Eye of the Storm: The Epidemiological Construction of AIDS.' Eds Elizabeth Fee and Daniel Fox. *AIDS: The Burdens of History*. Berkeley: University of California Press, 1988. 267–300.

——. 'Causes, Cases and Cohorts: The Role of Epidemiology in the Historical Construction of AIDS.' Eds Elizabeth Fee and Daniel Fox. *AIDS: The Making of a Chronic Disease*. Berkeley: University of California Press, 1992. 49–83.

Ostergard, Robert Jr 'Politics in the Hot Zone: AIDS and National Security in Africa.' *Third World Quarterly* 23.2 (2002): 335–50.

Owoh, Kenna, *World Bank Investing in Health: Is This All There Is*. Conference paper. Hofstra University Conference *The United Nations at Fifty*. 15–18 Mar. 1995.

Oxfam International. *Final Doha Declaration: Victory on Public Health but Few Other Gains for People in Poverty*. Press release. 14 Nov. 2001.

Oxfam International. *HIV/AIDS and Food Insecurity in Southern Africa*. 1 Dec. 2002 (http://www.oxfam.org/eng/pdfs/pp0211127_aids_safrica.pdf).

Patton, Cindy. *Inventing AIDS*. London: Routledge, 1990.

Pela, A. Ona, and Jerome J. Platt. 'AIDS in Africa: Emerging Trends.' *Social Science and Medicine* 28.1 (1989): 1–8.

Pettifor, Ann. 'Debt Cancellation, Lender Responsibility and Poor Country Empowerment.' *Review of African Political Economy* 27.83 (Mar. 2000): 138–45.

Piot, Peter. 'Heterosexual Transmission of HIV.' *AIDS* 1 (1997): 199–206.

Plumley, B., P. Bery, and C. Dadd. 'Beyond the Workplace: Business Participation in the Multi-sectoral Response to HIV/AIDS.' Conference paper. XIV International Conference on AIDS. Barcelona: July 2002.

Poku, N. K. 'The Global AIDS Fund: Context and Opportunity.' *Third World Quarterly* 23.2 (Apr. 2002): 283–98.

——. 'Poverty, Debt and Africa's HIV/AIDS Crisis.' *International Affairs* 78.3 (2002): 531–46.

——. 'The Global AIDS Fund: Context and Opportunity.' *Third World Quarterly* 23.2 (2002): 283–98.

Powesland, P. G. 'History of the Migration in Uganda.' Ed. Audrey Richards. *Economic Development and Tribal Change: A Study of Immigrant Labour in Buganda*. Cambridge: W. Heffer and Sons, 1952. 17–51.

Pretty, Jules. 'Can Sustainable Agriculture Feed Africa? New Evidence on Progress, Processes, and Impact.' *Environment, Development and Sustainability* 1 (1999): 253–74.

Price-Smith, Andrew. 'The HIV/AIDS Pandemic as a Threat to Governance and National Security: The Case of South Africa.' Conference paper. ISA Annual conference. Portland: Feb. 2003.

Rankin, Katharine N. 'Governing Development: Neoliberalism, Microcredit and Rational Economic Woman.' *Economy and Society* 30.1 (Feb. 2001): 18–37.

Revill, Jo. 'How Africa Can Win the Battle against AIDS.' *Guardian Weekly* 31 July–6 Aug. 2003.

Rhomushuna, Dr J. (Commisioner of Research for UAC). Personal Communication. Sept. 1992.

Richards, Audrey, ed. *Economic Development and Tribal Change: A Study of Immigrant Labour in Buganda.* Cambridge: W. Heffer and Sons, 1952.

——. 'The Travel Routes and the Travellers.' Ed. Audrey Richards. *Economic Development and Tribal Change: A Study of Immigrant Labour in Buganda.* Cambridge: W. Heffer and Sons, 1952. 52–76.

Robertson, Claire and Iris Berger, eds. *Women and Class in Africa.* New York: Holmes and Meier, 1986.

Robinson, J. *Prescription Games.* Toronto: McClelland and Stewart, 2001.

Robinson, Mark. 'Privatising the Voluntary Sector: NGOs as Public Service Contractors?' Eds David Hulme and Michael Edwards. *NGOs, States and Donors: Too Close for Comfort?* New York: St Martin's Press, 1997. 59–78.

Roscoe, John. *Twenty-five Years in East Africa.* Cambridge: Cambridge University Press, 1921.

Rose, Warner. 'The US Special 301 Process.' US Department of State: International Information Program (http://USinfo.state.gov/products/pubs/intelprop/301.htm)

Rosen, Sydney and Jonathon Simon. 'Shifting the Burden: The Private Sector's Response to the AIDS Epidemic in Africa.' *Bulletin of the World Health Organization* 81.2 (2003): 131–37.

Rugalema, Gabriel. 'Coping or Struggling? A Journey into the Impact of HIV/AIDS in Southern Africa.' *Review of African Political Economy*, 28.86 (2000): 537–45.

Sacks, Karen. *Sisters and Wives: The Past and Future of Sexual Equality.* Chicago: University of Illinois Press, 1982.

Sager, Alan and Deborah Socolar. 'Drug Industry Marketing Staff Soars While Research Staffing Stagnates.' *RxPolicy* (6 Dec. 2001) (http://rxpolicy.com/studies/bu-rxpromotion-v-randd.pdf).

Salleh, Ariel. *Ecofeminism as Politics: Nature, Marx and the Postmodern.* London: Zed Books, 1997.

Save the Children Fund. *Enumeration and Needs Assessment of Orphans in Uganda.* Unpublished report prepared for the Department of Social Rehabilitation. Kampala: SCF/Makerere University, 1991.

Scheper-Hughes, Nancy. 'AIDS and the Social Body.' *Social Science and Medicine* 39 (1994): 991–1003.

Scherer, F. M. and Jayashree Watal. 'Post-TRIPS Options for Access to Patented Medicines in Developing Nations.' *Journal of International Economic Law* (2002): 913–39.

Schiller, Laurence. 'The Royal Women of Buganda.' *The International Journal of African Historical Studies* 23.3 (1990): 453–73.

Schoepf, Brooke G. 'Ethical, Methodological and Political Issues of AIDS Research in Central Africa.' *Social Science and Medicine* 33.7 (1991): 749–63.

——. 'Action Research on Women in Kinshasa: Community-Based Risk Reduction Support.' Unpublished paper. 1992.

——. 'Political Economy, Sex and Cultural Logics: A View from Zaire.' *African Urban Quarterly* 6.1/2 (1991): 94–106.

Schoepf, Brooke G., Claude Schoepf, and Joyce Millen. 'Theoretical Therapies, Remote Remedies: SAPs and the Political Ecology of Poverty and Health in Africa.' Eds Jim Schopper, Doris and Serge Doussantousse. 'Sexual Behaviours Relevant to HIV Transmission in a Rural African Population: How Much Can a KAP Survey Tell Us?' Unpublished paper. Kampala: MSF, Oct. 1991.

Seeley, J. *et al.* 'The Extended Family and Support for People with AIDS in a Rural Population in South West Uganda: A Safety Net with Holes?' *AIDS Care* 5.1 (1993): 117–22.

Seidel, Gill. 'The Competing Discourses of HIV/AIDS in Sub-Saharan Africa: Discourses of Rights and Empowerment vs Discourses of Exclusion.' *Social Science and Medicine.* 36.3 (1993): 175–94.

——. 'Women at Risk: Gender and AIDS in Africa.' *Disasters* 17.2 (1993): 133–42.

Serwadda, D. 'Slim Disease: A New Disease in Uganda and its Association with HTLV-III Infection.' *The Lancet* 19 (1985): 849–52.

Sewankambo, Nelson and Dennis Willms. 'Promoting Sexual Health in Lyantonde, Uganda: A Participatory Action Research (PAR) Proposal.' Submission to IDRC, July 1995.

Sewankambo, Nelson *et al.* 'Demographic Impact of HIV Infection in Rural Rakai District, Uganda: Results of a Population-based Cohort Study.' *AIDS* 8.2 (1994): 1707–13.

Singer, Peter. *One World: The Ethics of Globalization.* New Haven: Yale University Press, 2002.

Singer, P. W. 'AIDS and International Security.' *Survival* 44 (2002): 145–58.

Solderholm, Peter and Roger Coate. *Institutionalized Chaos: AIDS, Environment and World Politics.* Conference paper. 34th Annual Meeting of the ISA. Mexico, Mar. 1993.

Southhall, A. W. and P. C. Gutkind. *Townsmen in the Making: Kampala and Its Suburbs.* Kampala: East African Institute of Social Research, 1957.

Stamp, Patricia. *Technology, Gender and Power in Africa.* Ottawa: IDRC Publications, 1990.

Starr, Paul. *The Social Transformation of American Medicine.* New York: Basic Books, 1982.

Steans, Jill. 'The Private is Global: Feminist Politics and Global Political Economy.' *New Political Economy* 4.1 (1999): 113–28.

Stewart, Sheelagh. 'Happily Ever After in the Marketplace: NGOs and Uncivil Society.' *Review of African Political Economy* 24.71 (1997): 11–34.

Stiglitz, Joseph E. *Globalization and its Discontents*. New York: W.W. Norton, 2002.

Stillwaggon, Eileen. 'HIV/AIDS in Africa: Fertile Terrain.' *Journal of Development Studies* 38.6 (2002): 1–22.

Strom, Stephanie. 'Gates Aims Billions to Attack Illnesses of World's Neediest.' *New York Times* 13 July 2003.

Summers, Carol. 'Intimate Colonialism: The Imperial Production of Reproduction in Uganda, 1907–1925.' *Signs* 16.4 (1991): 787–807.

Szeftel, Morris. 'Editorial: Globalization and African Responses.' *Review of African Political Economy* 27.85 (2000): 353–57.

Tan-Torres Edejer, Tessa. 'Health for Some: Health, Poverty, and Equity at the Beginning of the 21st Century.' Eds Victor Neufeld and Nancy Johnson. *Forging Links for Health Research: Perspectives from the Council on Health Research for Development*. Ottawa: IDRC, 2001.

TASO. 'Living Positively with AIDS: The AIDS Support Organization (TASO) Uganda.' No. 2, Strategies for Hope Series, 1991.

Taylor, Ian and Philip Nel. ' "New Africa," Globalization and the Confines of Elite Reform: "Getting the Rhetoric Right," Getting the Strategy Wrong.' *Third World Quarterly* 23.1 (2002): 163–80.

Taylor, Thomas. 'The Establishment of a European Plantation Sector Within the Emerging Colonial Economy of Uganda, 1902–1919.' *International Journal of African Historical Studies* 19.1 (1986): 35–58.

Tembo, George *et al*. 'Bed Occupancy due to HIV/AIDS in an Urban Hospital Medical Ward in Uganda.' *AIDS* 8.8 (1994): 1169–71.

't Hoen, Ellen. 'Globalization and Equitable Access to Essential Drugs.' *Third World Network* (Aug.–Sept. 2000) (http://www.twnside.org.sg/title/twr120c.htm).

Thomas, Caroline. 'Trade Policy and the Politics of Access to Drugs.' *Third World Quarterly* 23.2 (2002): 251–64.

Thompson, Carol. 'Regional Challenges to Globalization: Perspectives from Southern Africa.' *New Political Economy* 5.1 (2002): 41–58.

Topouzis, Daphne. 'Uganda: The Socio-economic Impact of HIV/AIDS on Rural Families with an Emphasis on Youth.' Rome: FAO, Feb. 1994.

Trachtman, Joel P. 'Legal Aspects of a Poverty Agenda at the WTO: Trade Law and Global Apartheid.' *Journal of International Economic Law* 6.1 (2003): 3–21.

Transnational Resource and Action Centre. *Tangled up in Blue: Corporate Partnerships at the United Nations*. Corporate Watch, Sept. 2002.

Treatment Action Campaign. 'TAC: An Overview.' (http://www.tac.org.za/Documents/Other/tachist.pdf).

Treichler, Paula. 'AIDS, Gender and Biomedical Discourse: Current Contests for Meaning.' Eds Elizabeth Fee and Daniel Fox. *AIDS: The Burden of History*. Los Angeles: University of California Press, 1998. 190–266.

Turshen, Meredith. 'US Aid to AIDS in Africa.' Eds George Bond *et al. AIDS in Africa and the Caribbean*. Boulder: Westview Press, 1997.

Tvedt, Terje. *Angels of Mercy or Development Diplomats? NGOs and Foreign Aid*. Oxford: James Currey, 1998.

Uganda AIDS Commission. 'Draft Mission Statement and Plan of Action for 1991/92.' Unpublished. Kampala: 1991.

——. 'Activity Inventory of ACPs in Uganda: Draft Document.' Unpublished. Kampala: 1992.

Uganda AIDS Commission Secretariat. *Uganda National Operational Plan for HIV/AIDS/STD Prevention, Care and Support, 1994–1998*. Kampala, 1993.

Uganda AIDS Commission Secretariat, *AIDS Control in Uganda: The Multisectoral Approach*. Unpublished. Kampala: 1993.

Uganda AIDS Commission Secretariat/UNAIDS. *The National Strategic Framework for HIV/AIDS Activities in Uganda 2000/1–2005/6*. 11 Nov. 2000.

Uganda AIDS Control Programme. *Medium-Term Plan for AIDS Control and Prevention*. WHO/Uganda Ministry of Health, 1986.

Uganda AIDS Control Programme/Ministry of Health. *Review of Uganda's ACP*. Dec. 1988.

Uganda ACP/MOH. *Progress Report on ACP 1 Jan. to 31 Apr. 1992*. Entebbe: Government Printers, 1992.

Uganda ACP/MOH/GPA. *An Evaluation of Uganda ACP's IEC Activities*. Unpublished draft report. Dec. 1991.

Uganda STD/AIDS Control Programme/Ministry of Health. *HIV/AIDS Surveillance Report Mar. 1996*. Entebbe: Government Printers, 1996.

Ulin, Patricia. 'African Women and AIDS: Negotiating Behavioral Change.' *Social Science and Medicine* 34.1 (1992): 63–73.

UNAIDS. 'Progress Report on the Development of a UN System Strategic Plan for HIV/AIDS 2001–2005.' UNAIDS/PCB(10)/ 00.5 (6 Nov. 2000).

——. 'Focus: AIDS and Human Rights.' *Report on the Global HIV/AIDS Epidemic 2002*. UNAIDS, 2002. 62–69 (http://www.unaids.org/barcelona/presskit/barcelona%20report/focus_humanrights.pdf).

——. *UNAIDS Partnership: Working Together on AIDS*. Geneva: May 2002.

——. *AIDS Epidemic Update*. Geneva: Dec. 2002.

——. 'HIV/AIDS and Security.' Fact sheet 1 (http://www.unaids.org/security/Information/Factsheets/FSI security.html).

——. 'Programme Coordinating Board Fourteenth Meeting Geneva, 26–27 June 2003, Decisions, Recommendations and Conclusions.' UNAIDS/PCB(14)/03.8 RECS.

UNAIDS *et al.* 'Accelerating Access to HIV/AIDS Care and Treatment in Developing Countries: A Joint Statement of Intent.' UNAIDS, 8 May 2000.

UNAIDS Secretariat. 'Accelerating Access to HIV/AIDS Care, Treatment and Support.' Progress Report Updated Nov. 2001.

UNAIDS Secretariat. *Mobilizing Billions to Fight AIDS in Africa: The Way Forward*. Geneva: n.d.

UNAIDS/FAO. 'HIV/AIDS Epidemic is Shifting from Cities to Rural Areas: New Focus on Agricultural Policy Needed.' Press release. Rome-Geneva: 22 June 2000.

UNAIDS/Programme Coordinating Board (9)/00.4. Geneva: UNAIDS, May 2000.

UNAIDS/UNICEF/WHO. 'Epidemiological Fact Sheet on HIV/AIDS and STIs.' Uganda: 2002.

UNDP. *Human Development Report 2003*. New York: Oxford UP, 2003.

UNICEF. Discussion Paper Towards the Development of UNICEF-Uganda Anti-AIDS Strategy. Kampala, Nov. 1991.

——. New Phase of UNICEF Support for AIDS Control in Uganda: Safeguard Youth from AIDS. Kampala: 1992.

——. 'An Evaluation of SYFA Programme.' Kampala: UNICEF/Uganda AIDS Commission, Nov. 1995.

'Update: UNAIDS Gets Swedish Support.' *AIDS and Society* 6.4 (July/Aug. 1995): 9.

Vaughan, Megan. *Curing their Ills: Colonial Power and African Illness*. Stanford: Stanford UP, 1991.

Vink, Annemieke. 'Coping Strategies among AIDS-Affected People in Kisoro District, Southwest Uganda.' Unpublished report prepared for the St Frances Hospital. Mutolere, Kisoro: 1996.

Watkins, Kevin. 'Eight Broken Promises: Why the WTO isn't Working for the World's Poor.' Oxfam Briefing Paper No. 9. Oxfam International, 2001.

Watney, Simon. *Practices of Freedom: Selected Writings on HIV/AIDS*. London: Meuthen, 1994.

Weissman, Robert. 'AIDS Drugs for Africa.' *Multinational Monitor* 20.9 (1999): 1–8.

Wellman, Sandra, *Kampala Women Getting by: Wellbeing in the Time of AIDS*. London: James Currey, 1996.

Werner, David. 'The Life and Death of PHC.' *Third World Resurgence* 42/43 (1994): 10–15.

White, Luise. *The Comforts of Home: Prostitution in Colonial Nairobi*. Chicago: University of Chicago Press, 1991.

White, Michael A. 'Talking About AIDS: The Biography of a Local AIDS Organization within the Church of Uganda.' Conference paper. 38th Annual Meeting of the African Studies Association. Orlando, Florida: Nov. 1995.

Whiteside, Alan. 'Poverty and HIV/AIDS in Africa.' *Third World Quarterly* 23.2 (2002): 313–32.

WHO. *Evaluation of Health Care for All by the Year 2000*. Geneva, 1987.

——. *Guidelines for the Development of a National AIDS Prevention and Control Programme*. Geneva: 1998.

——. 'Impact of AIDS on Older People in Africa.' Geneva: WHO, Dec. 2002 (http://www.who.int/hpr/ageing/zimaidsreport.pdf).

——. 'What are "Intellectual Property Rights?" ' *Frequently Asked Questions about TRIPS* (http://www.wto.org/english/tratop_e/trips_e/tripfq_ehtm# WhatAre).

——. *WHO Model List 13th Edition*. Apr. 2003 (http://www.who.int/medicines/organization/par/edl/expcom13/eml13_en.pdf).

WHO/GPA. *Report of the External Review of the World Health Organization Global Programme on AIDS* GPA/GMC (8)92.4. Geneva: Jan. 1997.

World Bank. 'About MAP.' (http:/ /www.worldbank.org/afr/aids/map.htm).

World Bank. *Sub-Saharan Africa: From Crisis to Sustainable Government*. Washington: The World Bank, 1989.

——. *World Development Report 1991: The Challenge of Development*. New York: Oxford University Press, 1991.

——. *Tanzania: AIDS Assessment and Planning Study*. Washington, World Bank, 1992.

——. *Uganda: Growing Out of Poverty*. Washington, D.C.: World Bank, 1993.

——. *Uganda Social Sector Strategy*. 1993.

——. *World Development Report 1993: Investing in Health*. New York: Oxford University Press, 1993.

——. *Action for Better Health in Africa: Executive Summary of the World Bank Publication Better Health in Africa*. Washington: World Bank 1994.

——. *Preparing and Implementing MAP Support to HIV/AIDS Country Programs in Africa: Guidelines and Lessons Learned*. Third Draft. 25 June 2002.

——. 'Poverty Eradication Through Improved Economic Growth, Governance, and Partnership: The Way Forward.' Kampala: Uganda Country Office, 14–16 May 2003.

World Bank, Uganda Country Office. *Poverty Eradication through Improved Economic Growth, Governance, and Partnership: The Way Forward*. Kampala, 14–16 May 2003.

Wrigley, Christopher. 'Four Steps Toward Disaster.' Eds H. B. Hansen and M. Twaddle. *Uganda Now: Between Decay and Development*. London: James Currey, 1988.

WTO/WHO. *WTO Agreements and Public Health: A Joint Study by the WHO and the WTO Secretariat*. WHO, 2002.

WTO. 'Declaration on the TRIPS Agreement and Public Health.' WTO Ministerial Conference 4th session. Doha: 9–14 Nov. 2001. WT/MIN(01)/DEC/W/2.

Yong Kim, J. *et al.*, eds. *Dying for Growth: Global Inequality and the Health of the Poor*. Monroe: Common Courage Press, 2000.

Young, Sherilynn. 'Fertility and Famine: Women's Agricultural History in Southern Mozambique.' Eds Robin Palmer and Neil Parsons. *The Roots of Rural Poverty in Central and Southern Africa*. Berkeley: University of California Press, 1977. 66–81.

Zuniga, J. 'Out of Africa: Uganda and AIDS.' *Journal of the International Association of Physicians in AIDS Care* (Oct. 1999): 1–12.

Index